The Wounding
of
Health Care

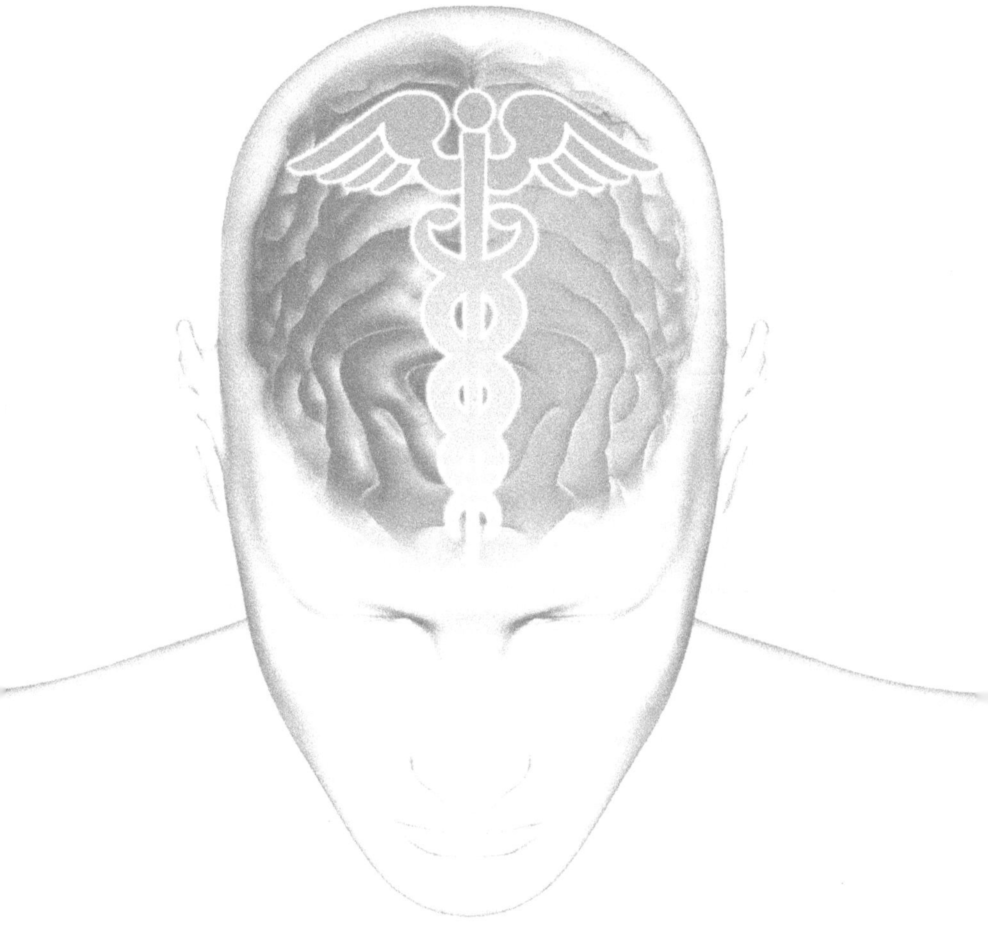

Published in Australia by
Opame Media
P.O. Box 7286, Karingal Centre, Frankston, VIC, 3199, Australia
Tel: +61 412 630 112
Email: catherinefyans@gmail.com
Website: www.catherinefyans.com / www.thewoundingofhealthcare.com

First published in Australia 2016
SECOND EDITION 2019
Copyright © Catherine Fyans 2016

All rights reserved. No part of this publication may be reproduced, stored in a retrieval system, or transmitted, in any form or by any means without the prior written permission of the publisher, nor be otherwise circulated in any form of binding or cover other than that in which it is published and without a similar condition being imposed on the subsequent purchaser.

 A catalogue record for this book is available from the National Library of Australia

National Library of Australia Cataloguing–in–Publication entry

Creator: Fyans, Catherine J., Author
Title: The Wounding of Health Care: From Fragmentation to Integration/ Catherine J. Fyans
ISBN: 978-0-9925163-1-4 (paperback)
Subjects: Medical care, Mind and body therapies
Other Creators/Contributors: Spedding, Amanda, Editor
Dewey Number: 362.1

Cover design by Nitsua
Typesetting by Nelly Murariu at PixBeeDesign.com
Printed by Createspace

Disclaimer
All care has been taken in the preparation of the information herein, but no responsibility can be accepted by the publisher or author for any damages resulting from the misinterpretation of this work. All contact details given in this book were current at the time of publication, but are subject to change.

The advice given in this book is based on the experience of the individuals. Professionals should be consulted for individual problems. The author and publisher shall not be responsible for any person with regard to any loss or damage caused directly or indirectly by the information in this book.

The Wounding *of* Health Care

From Fragmentation to Integration

Dr Catherine J. Fyans

The Wounding *of* Health Care

From Fragmentation to Integration

Dr Catherine J. Fyans

*For Marcus and Daniel.
Thank you for bringing me back to
what is really important in life.*

Disclaimer

Though Dr Fyans is a health-care professional, this book is in no way aimed to give specific medical advice. Though there might be some guidelines and suggestions throughout the book, it is designed to give an overview of health care as she sees it, and to maybe stimulate debate and inquiry. She recommends that any individual address their personal health-care concerns with their own health-care practitioners.

All case studies in this book have been blended and have had names and details changed so as to not identify any individuals. The comments regarding the mind-body connection of specific medical conditions are generalisations and might not apply to all individuals who have these conditions. It should be understood that despite general trends and patterns there are many individual variations regarding illness causation and manifestation.

Dr Fyans does not represent any group in her comments and opinions.

Contents

Acknowledgements	11
Introduction	13
Prologue	19
Chapter 1 | Emotions and Health	21
Chapter 2 | Consciousness	55
Chapter 3 | Energy Medicine	91
Chapter 4 | Beliefs	121
Chapter 5 | Stress	133
Chapter 6 | From Victimhood to Empowerment in Health	157
Chapter 7 | The Meaning of Illness	195
Chapter 8 | Love versus Fear in Health Care	243
Chapter 9 | From a Physician's Perspective	261
Epilogue – 'White Christmas'	285
About the Author	293

Acknowledgements

I am immensely grateful to publishing consultant, Julie Postance, for her expert and encouraging advice and guidance, and for the many times that she patiently dissuaded me from throwing my manuscript 'in the bin'.

Many thanks to Amanda Spedding, for her professional and seamless handling of my manuscript, and to Cornelia Murariu for her artistry and precision. It was a great comfort for me to know that my manuscript was in such good hands.

I thank Wendy Hastrich and Jenni Wadsworth for their honest evaluation of my manuscript, and Ben Hannah for his insightful advice and support.

Over countless years, I have been very fortunate to have had numerous expert mentors and teachers, too many to name. I thank them all for their tireless enthusiasm and generosity in teaching their vast knowledge and finely-honed skills.

I am blessed to have my two wonderful sons, Marcus and Daniel, in my life. I thank them for their unconditional support, and for keeping me grounded and 'real'. So proud to be their mother!

And thank you to 'Life' – though we have sometimes had a fraught relationship – I am humbled and grateful for the many lessons that you persistently and lovingly provide me with, and that have fuelled the writing of this book.

Introduction

This book is more about posing questions than giving answers. It is my 'talking out loud' and trying to summarise my questions regarding health care, and life in general (as they are not separate), that have perplexed and intrigued me for many years. Sometimes we do not ask "why?" often enough. We are so conditioned and so accepting of the way things are that we rarely step outside the status quo to have a look inside. The biggest question I pose is: "What actually *is* healing?"

I am in no way representative of any of the health professional or other groups I have been involved with. I stand alone in what I have to say and share. No-one has the full answer to life's dilemmas, including health issues, for anyone else. This book is not designed to give any specific medical advice and I recommend that you discuss any of your personal health and wellbeing concerns with your own health-care professionals.

My writings present my own individual perspective. It will be different to anyone else's perspective as none of us see life in quite the same way even though we have many agreed-upon, commonly-held perceptions. This is a very subjective book, and is not backed by objective measurement and data. There is no 'proof' in these pages. I have written it as I see it. I do not want anyone to agree with my version of reality and how I see the practise of health care. I would, however, hope my comments might help you to have a good look at, and question, whether all current systems and practises are for your benefit.

My natural tendency is to look at the overview rather than the details. I have also had a tendency to stand on the outside, looking into and observing a situation or group rather than being fully immersed within it – more of a loner than a group player you could say. And that has been both painful and beneficial in that I rarely feel I fully belong to a group, yet have gained a perspective that I think others might not.

This is not a 'how to do' book, though there is some splattering of suggestions throughout it. Let me repeat – this is not a 'how to do' book. You will not find any diagrams, illustrations, graphs or research findings here. There are many esteemed authors who have already done this very well, and I would not attempt to emulate them. My own experience and observations largely contribute to the writing of this book.

I do respect science and the great benefits to humanity that have been derived from it; however, I also love a bit of mystery and secretly hope we do not find the answers to all phenomena. And I do not think we will, as 'Life' is ever evolving and, I expect, will be forever a step ahead of our intellectual understanding. I do hope mystery and science meet to develop a happy and respectful relationship, and share with each other the best of themselves. I am encouraged that this seems to be happening.

My observations gleaned from many years of working with people and their myriad problems, in addition to my own life experience, contribute largely to the writing of this book. I make no apologies for using myself as one of the people being observed, though we can never fully observe ourselves. I write this book from the position that I am well and truly in the throng of our shared humanity. Your life challenges are my life challenges. Your story is my story – we are one.

Regarding the case studies I have included in the book, I have changed all names and I have blended 'cases' so as to not identify or isolate any individual. The intent is not to personalise the cases, though they might seem very personal, but to look at trends I have observed in a large number of people over many years. So if you are reading this and you think it is you – it is not! There is a lot of commonality in what we all experience, and I can personally, at some level, identify with most of what I have observed in others and have thus written about.

I am immensely grateful for the many people I have been privileged to call 'my patients'. I have learnt so much from all of you and I thank you for trusting me enough to share your rich life journeys with me. Life on Earth is not always easy and I am amazed at what the human spirit can endure and grow through. You are all heroes in my eyes.

I am very blessed to have been trained in both the worlds of conventional Western medicine and 'alternative' and energy medicine. Bundled together I like to call it 'integrative' medicine. I can speak the language of chakras as well as speak the language of biochemistry. I can easily slip from one paradigm to the other, as I know they are not really separate but just different manifestations and interpretations of the one universal energy. From the bottom of my heart I thank all of my teachers and mentors who have guided me on this journey. You are also my heroes.

I have a long-standing and passionate interest in 'mind-body' medicine, particularly in the subconscious influences on physical and psychological health. My interest in this area was ignited when I worked with Tibetan refugees in North India in the mid-1980s, and was there exposed to another world-view, which, for me, challenged many of the dogmas that were instilled during my medical training. That experience, in many ways, was pivotal in my wanting to look beyond current belief-systems and ways of doing things. You could say I have been on a steady search since – almost 30 years, of trying to understand health and healing from many different perspectives.

I am very aware of the force of our beliefs, especially when they are shared by the majority; of how they are hard-wired into our collective consciousness and into our physical lives and understandings of health as a result. When the whole structure of our health-care system is aligned with collective beliefs, it is an enormous and risky task to try to affect change. But one has to start somewhere and it is evolutionary, and maybe revolutionary, to do so. I applaud the many people who are on their missions to do so.

Change happens – it is an inevitable part of life; but what can appear to be significant change often happens within the confines of an unchanging paradigm. Change is really about changing understandings and concepts, and thus beliefs. It is about evolution and growth; about learning from, but letting go of things from the past that no longer serve us. Part of our evolution is to question current systems and ways of doing things and explore new concepts and ways of being. This is part of our job description – to evolve. Society wants us to be compliant. It suits many people to not question what we currently, commonly accept as truth.

I write a lot about emotions and psychological considerations in this book. You might well ask: "What has that got to do with health?" And my answer is: "Everything." I do not and cannot separate mind from body, even though that is still the prevailing belief-system of the profession in which I work. The belief in body being separate from mind has never made any sense to me. I believe the physical aspects we experience as health issues are downward manifestations of what we hold in mind. Prevention is better than cure, so addressing the underlying mind-related causes might go a long way in preventing the physical effects we call illness.

Having worked in health care in a number of different situations for over 35 years has given me a long time to observe the prevailing systems. I have worked primarily in Western medicine (my 'day job') but have also studied, or been exposed to, many other healing disciplines including kinesiology, psychosomatic medicine, medical intuition, shamanic healing methods and many others. My curiosity, and probably my gullibility, has led me down many and varied paths, some from which I made a very hasty retreat, and some that have gifted me enormously with a fountain of knowledge and understandings.

Because of an insatiable curiosity, and wanting to find the best healing methods available, I have a fair insight into a variety of approaches to, and philosophies about, health care. Probably, though, there are many others I have not yet been acquainted with. They all have their merits and limitations. Though my main training and main work has been in Western, allopathic medicine, I consider myself an individual and choose not to be defined by, or limited to, any one group.

My dream is that the different health-care disciplines truly complement each other; each offering their areas of expertise for the overall benefit of the health-care consumer and practitioner – each acknowledging their own and the others' skills in an atmosphere of positive exchange and learning. I look forward to a time when we have this cooperative, win-win system. This is what true 'integrative' health care should be about – and why not?

I believe in the patient/client being their own authority, as best they can; with the health-care practitioner being the advisor and facilitator. It is time for the power and authority to be given back to the client. I believe education is a crucial part of health care. As the Chinese proverb states: 'Give a man a fish and he will eat for a day. Teach a man to fish and he will eat for the rest of his life.'

I have been very blessed to sit at the feet of many masters (sometimes literally!). I have been taught by some of the best mind-body medicine experts on the planet; some very well-known and others who truly 'fly under the radar'; some through their writings, lectures, teachings and workshops; some in person, some from afar. I am sure there must be many more who I have not met, read about, or even heard of as yet. I thank you all for the great gifts that you share with humankind and for your courage, tenacity, intelligence, compassion, wisdom and vision in the sharing of these. I bow in reverence to who you are and what you do.

Having, like everyone, been presented with my fair share of challenges in life I have had to do the 'hard yards' in looking at and healing my own issues. This is definitely a work in progress! I have personally had to deal with much of what I write about – same triumphs and issues. How could it be otherwise? I have had many personal experiences that have pushed me to try to find some answers, in addition to having the responsibility of needing to help others deal with their own challenges.

We are all entitled to our own opinions and beliefs; the question is not whether they are good or bad, accurate or not, but whether they are beneficial in terms of our individual and collective happiness and evolution. I would highly suggest you take from this what you might find beneficial, or at least interesting, and leave the rest. You be the judge of what resonates with you.

An interesting aspect of writing a book is knowing that what one is currently sharing will be inevitably upgraded over time; in some cases even before the original book is completed. This is because our individual and collective understandings and beliefs inevitably change as part of our evolution. On the other hand, what we put out to share will be part of what influences change, one way or another. The truth of the moment may, or may not, be the truth of the future.

My personal life experience has been my greatest learning. I do believe that *Life* is the greatest teacher there is. Trust it and yourself!

Prologue

I had a dream many years ago. It was one of those very vivid dreams that are still clearly remembered many years later. In the dream I was a street-wise male youth of about 16. The setting was a town that appeared to be somewhere in Europe. It felt very familiar, though I do not recall having visited such a place in my non-dream state. I was alone but amongst a group of civilians who were terrorised by, and fleeing from, some sort of military-like, malevolent group. There was great fear and mayhem and a potent atmosphere of oppression.

I found myself running from an older male who was one of the oppressors. He appeared to be in some sort of uniform and was an austere and frightening figure. He was very determined to catch me. I was fast but so was he. I found myself running into a house with my pursuer hot on my heels. The house was narrow, nestled amongst a group of similar houses, and had a number of floors.

I ran up the stairs in terror until I reached a room on the top floor. I tried to close the door but it was forced open and the man entered. It was a small, unfurnished room with a window opposite the door. I had my back to the window and the man approached with a small object held in his right hand. He thrust his hand forward, holding the object between his index finger and thumb, pushing it in front of my face in a threatening manner. It was a small medicine-like capsule with a hook – similar to fishhook – inside it.

As he lunged towards me, being a fit and agile youth, I managed to manoeuvre my way to the side and used his momentum to tip him through the open window. He fell three floors to the ground and I jumped after him, landing on his body. I then grabbed a large rock that was lying nearby and hit him on the head with it to make sure he was indeed dead. I then ran off to join the other fleeing civilians.

What was this dream, that I still remember so well many years later, trying to tell me? The sense was that the forcing, controlling system, represented by the man in uniform, depicted the worst aspects of the modern health-care system; the aspects based on fear, rigid rules and regulations, and force. These aspects do not allow health-care practitioners, and health-care consumers alike, to have the freedom to use their own knowing and intuition to guide them in matters of health.

The hook in the capsule depicted being hooked, or forced, into abeyance to a system that promotes the 'cure' from the outside, usually in the form of chemicals, rather than providing people with education to encourage them to use their own minds to activate the healing power from within. My killing the military man (and I was going to leave that part out – but for the sake of honesty…) represented my personal and life-long interest in helping to shift some beliefs regarding health care that, in my opinion, no longer serve us well.

Chapter 1

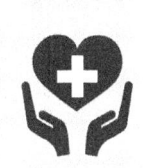

Emotions and Health

"I wish I could show you when you are lonely or in darkness the astonishing light of your own being."

HAFIZ OF SHIRAZ

It was a busy, hot day at the skin cancer clinic. About halfway through the afternoon shift I entered the consulting room to see yet another of the many patients scheduled for that afternoon. Alfred had come in for his routine yearly skin check. He was an elderly man with a gentle nature. Maria, the nurse, had already efficiently tended to the preliminary procedures.

During the examination I asked Alfred a few general questions to help personalise what can seem like a very impersonal process. I had noted that he looked sad and his eyes filled with tears as he mentioned he was grieving the loss of his little dog that had died some weeks earlier. For years, the little dog had been this man's main companion, maybe only companion, and he was acutely feeling her absence.

Maria and I could not say much to comfort him, nor did we try; but we paused what we were doing and listened to his expression of grief, for we both knew that as he lived alone and did not have family, this might be the only opportunity for him to do so.

I was struck by the almost child-like innocence and purity of his expression. As is so often the case, the three of us being in that room at that time was not just about his skin examination, it was about taking that brief opportunity to allow another human being to express his emotional pain in an atmosphere of acceptance and empathy.

In the above example, we could not 'fix it' or make it right; and that is often not the point. It is when we are able to express our emotions in their pure, unadulterated form that they move through our system and release, rather than remain stuck and distorted. This applies to any emotion but our painful emotions are particularly relevant to this discussion, as these are the ones we are more likely to resist and suppress. The very awareness, and sometimes expression and release of emotions, starts their integration and transmutation to a higher form.

I unapologetically spend a large section of this book on emotional health. This is not so much from a psychological point of view as from a human point of view. My interest in emotions is more in how they affect our day-to-day life, and our health and wellbeing. I believe our physical health is intimately connected to our mental and emotional aspects. I am not focusing on psychopathology as that is out of the scope of this book and I do suggest that anyone with concerns in that area seek help from appropriately-trained professionals.

We engage and experience life through our emotions, and when we feel our emotions we better integrate our experiences. When we suppress our emotions we do not assimilate our experiences, nor gain insights from them. Put plainly, we are designed to feel. At a core level, our quality of life is determined by how we feel about ourselves, other people and life in general. Most, if not all, of what we do is motivated by wanting to feel better – even if what we do to that aim is sometimes awry. How we feel will lead us through the maze of life.

How we feel emotionally affects our moment-to-moment experience of life; and our experiences give rise to our emotions. How we handle our emotional life will have a potent effect on our wellbeing. It will also have a significant effect on those around us. Emotions are a means by which we connect with others and share this human experience. How we express our emotions will indicate to others, truthfully, our current state of being and level of development.

Emotions imprint our experiences. They give flavour and colour to what we live through. We interpret our experiences based on how we feel about them, and this in turn relates to what we have recorded from similar experiences in the past. How we feel related to a current situation can lead us to the beliefs and conclusions about life that we have formulated from our past. These beliefs and conclusions very much affect our physical health.

Terms such as 'emotional intelligence' and 'mindfulness' are now common parlance and have reached many sectors of society, as we, as a society, become more emotionally intelligent.

Some might argue that emotions follow thought; others believe that thought springs from emotions, or that they work together in a circular fashion feeding into and reinforcing each other. Some would put forward that emotions are the body's translation of thought into physical sensations and feelings. In accordance with the holographic view of reality, I believe that thoughts and emotions are concurrent and just different expressions of the same energy. But who knows, and does it matter? The bottom line is that how we *feel* – matters, and will affect our health and wellbeing.

Emotional Suppression

I had known Miranda for a number of years and saw her intermittently, mainly when she came for her yearly women's health check. Miranda was always beautifully groomed and dressed and I do not ever recall seeing her in the casual, comfortable clothes most of my patients wore. She balanced a demanding profession in the legal sector with raising a family, and appeared to do both very well. However, she indicated that she had some significant problems with some of her personal relationships and in her work life but had chosen to live with this, as she believed this situation was far better than any contemplated alternative. Though very pleasant, there was palpable tension about her and this reflected in her speech and her body language.

I never succeeded in drawing out the emotions I sensed were percolating under the surface. I would have been transgressing a boundary to have even tried, as there was a clear unvoiced message to not venture there. She acknowledged that all was not well in her life but had chosen to not change things and risk the upheaval this might entail. She was an intelligent woman and had made a conscious choice to not delve into the world of feeling nor look at the information those inner stirrings were trying to impart.

Over the years she was diagnosed with a number of illnesses, including a form of cancer. When I last saw her she was maintaining her usual work and lifestyle with little change, whilst looking frailer and taking a burgeoning list of medications.

I might use the words 'supressed' and 'repressed' interchangeably. My understanding is that 'suppression' is when we knowingly put a thought or feeling below conscious awareness – out of the way; and 'repression' is when the process is completely unconscious and thus the mind content more deeply hidden. The term 'emotion' is an objective description of what we are feeling as a visceral mind-body experience.

I have often pondered on how emotional suppression and repression can cause such havoc to our physiology. It seems like such a useful strategy at times, and is certainly condoned by large sectors of society! My simple understanding is that when we suppress/repress emotions we are blocking the life force, the natural flow of energies and the information these emotions are trying to impart. We are also fragmenting our experiences, and thus ourselves, by our non-integration of them.

Whatever we are feeling is the truth of the moment, regardless of whether we like it or not, and will indicate to us the flavour of our related thought-patterns. In fact that is the job of emotions – to give us a clue as to the underlying thought-patterns and beliefs we are holding on the subject at hand.

We cannot adjust and correct that of which we are unaware; and emotions are our indicators of the vibration of our thoughts and beliefs. Basically, how we feel is telling us something about our underlying thoughts, beliefs and attitudes related to a given situation; and these will not be addressed, and will thus perpetuate, if the related emotions are suppressed.

Some might argue that the suppression of emotions utilises considerably more energy than if they are allowed to flow. We might particularly suppress the emotions we, or others, have judged as 'bad', and for which we might have been punished in early life. For example, the emotion of anger is often disapproved of and punished. This often occurs in childhood, but also in later life when it is considered inappropriate and politically incorrect to express certain emotions in certain sectors of society. For some it might be considered appropriate, and for others not.

We are so preoccupied with judging emotions as 'good' or 'bad', 'positive' or 'negative'. Emotions are neither good nor bad, but always *accurate* in indicating to us – and others – our associated thought-patterns and conclusions about life. If we are trying to squash our anger, without upgrading our understandings and beliefs related to *why* that anger came about, we are taking the battery out of the alarm.

We need to be in touch with our living emotional centre to be guided by it. It is not the negative emotions that are the problem. It is our judging, and then suppressing or projecting them, that is far more harmful. Emotions, whether positive or negative, are just doing the job they are designed to do. They are designed to get our attention.

When we dull the capacity to feel, we dull the capacity to feel *all* emotions, including joy, and accordingly dampen our intuition and creative abilities. We also dull the capacity to tune into our position relative to our current circumstances, and this might include our capacity to create appropriate boundaries.

We can definitely suppress the happier emotions; however, we are more likely to suppress what we experience as painful. When our minds have cultivated the habit of not feeling emotional pain, it becomes more and more difficult to feel *any* emotion, and that door to our inner being can become firmly shut. The ploy to avoid feeling painful emotions simply does not work in the long run.

When we do not tune into our own feelings and emotions, it is difficult to tune into those of others. When someone has shut down their own feelings they cannot have a level of empathy for others and will act accordingly. Empathy is when we have a feeling-sense of what another is experiencing. At the extreme, emotional shut down and lack of empathy can give rise to cruelty and be the basis of psychopathy and evil.

Underlying this extreme is often unresolved deep wounding and pain experienced at an early age. The pain and related behaviours will then likely be transmitted down the generations, the wounding becoming trans-generational. We see families, organisations and whole societies subject to this dynamic of shutting down the spectrum of emotions and thus human warmth, compassion and empathy.

'Shock' is when we quickly suppress an emotion related to a situation we do not want to experience. We are resisting and shutting the experience out. This, of course, has its place, especially when we are young and do not have the capacity to handle what we might be exposed to. It can also happen when we are older. It is well understood that some situations are exceedingly difficult to bear; however, the more one goes into shock and suppression, the more one is likely to later carry those unresolved emotions as 'post-traumatic stress disorder' (PTSD) or similar.

This process of shock and suppression also has the potential to adversely affect our bodies, as the body might quickly translate and compensate for what the mind cannot handle. There will be a biological adaptation in an attempt to ensure survival, and this can contribute to illness manifestation. This is a deeply unconscious process. When we are able to deal emotionally with the situation at hand, we are less likely to suppress the emotions, which might later find on outlet as a physical or psychological disorder.

When you have been suppressing emotions you can feel the tension in your body. This might particularly occur when you are busy, distracted and not present with yourself. You might then coax these emotions gently to the fore when you know they are lurking in the background. Sometimes you might gain quick insights and clarity, and sometimes *life* will reliably help bring this about. When you maintain awareness of your emotional reactions and heed the information, they will come and go like ripples rather than tsunamis.

Emotional Release

Emotional release is not about wallowing in the emotions and perpetuating the related 'story', but about freeing up the energy and maturing the emotions. It is ultimately about changing what stimulated the emotional upset in the first place. Sometimes just the free and unexaggerated awareness and expression is all that is needed for their integration and maturation – just letting them come and go and move through our system naturally. Often the insights will flow when we allow this. (Note: this does not mean 'acting them out' or directing them towards another.)

In our society we have paid homage to the intellect, and the physical/material, at the expense of the emotional realm. We have been very good at honing our intellects and knowledge-base as well as putting value on the material aspects of life. We have viewed emotions as much less significant and less valuable. We have attached our egos and pride to what we know, what we achieve and what we own. Meanwhile, we have tended to individually and collectively cut ourselves off from our hearts. Ideally, the intellectual, physical and emotional realms work in harmony for balance of the individual and society as a whole.

Emotions will remain at the level of when they were suppressed or repressed despite intellectual prowess and maturity in other areas. Our immature, childish emotions are more likely to bring us pain and thus are the ones we are most likely to suppress in an attempt to avoid this pain. This might well be the best option at certain vulnerable points in our life, and especially when we do not have the ego strength to deal with them.

However, they will remain at the immature level of when they were suppressed, until brought into consciousness and *felt*, or until underlying beliefs and thought-patterns are adjusted. Insights will flow as we allow these emotions to be felt. They will then more likely naturally mature to a level beyond pain, and thus be transmuted. It is a matter of employing our intellectual understandings whilst allowing our suppressed emotions to be felt.

Feeling our emotions can feel like annihilation to the ego, so there can be a great deal of resistance to this. The resistance can be due to the discomfort of feeling the emotions themselves, but often more so from seeing oneself – in having these emotions – as not the idealised version we thought we were. We believe that feeling and expressing certain emotions is inconsistent with the image we might want to portray, and is threatening to our acceptance by, and thus survival in, our society. We conclude that the solution is to avoid feeling; thus we suppress these uncomfortable emotions.

The release of emotions cannot be just a cognitive process. The adage 'the healing is in the feeling' is very valid in my opinion. We cannot release an emotion by *thinking* it away, though we can *intend* that the process will happen, and in the best and easiest way possible. Emotions need to be *felt*, and life has a way of triggering those emotions if we allow it. In this sense, I believe that 'Life' is the best teacher we have. It knows when and how to trigger what needs to be brought into conscious awareness where it can be acknowledged and addressed.

The process of feeling our emotions will help highlight any underlying distortions in our beliefs and understandings of life. Pure emotions are honest. They will accurately indicate where we are on a subject, in the moment. We either feel good or we feel bad, indicating that our underlying thought-patterns and beliefs are beneficial to us or not.

Part of this process is just allowing those emotions to naturally come to the fore, and trusting that life has a way of bringing this about, rather than forcing them. There is a large difference between identifying and changing what we don't like about ourselves and covering, and thus suppressing, what we are rejecting. The mask just hides what we don't want to acknowledge in ourselves, which therefore will never truly be addressed – until some crisis (including illness) might impel us to do so.

Of course we need to use our frontal lobes and our intellects in this process. The aim is not to wallow in our emotions or unleash them in a harmful way but to hone our *awareness* of them and then use our intellects to adjust what triggered them in the first place. The truth is that when we let go of the resistance and truly allow ourselves to feel, we will gain more intellectual clarity as those emotions dissipate. They will control us less. This process can be very gentle and contained. It is not about uncontrolled expression. There is a fine line between *managing* our emotions and suppressing them.

Life is about experiencing a gamut of events, all ultimately for our growth and evolvement, and for better refining what we *do* want to experience and how we want to evolve. When we avoid feeling, which really means avoiding life experience in our attempt to avoid emotional discomfort, it can be akin to cheating life. 'Being out of your comfort zone' really means being willing to endure some uncomfortable emotions related to new or novel experiences and endeavours.

It has taken me many years to get to a point where I am more comfortable with how I genuinely feel, even though this might not fit the image I might want to portray. We have collectively decided that to display any sort of vulnerability is weak, immature and just shameful. It does not fit with the idealised images we feel we need to have to gain acceptance and approval from our communities, and thus survive in them.

We live in a very 'look at me' society. "Look at me. Look at me. But please do not look at the *real* me, for I believe you will judge what you see."

Trust in your own Imperfection

I have a large gap between my two front teeth, which reminds me of one of my imperfections on a daily basis. Not at all fashionable in this climate of expensively-aligned and whitened teeth, but there it is for all to see.

Like all of us, I have my share of flaws, issues, and neuroses. Through my imperfections I have experienced much of the spectrum of human sufferings and failings; and, just for the record, choose to not to cover the *whole* spectrum – thank you very much, 'Universe'! And through all of this I have maybe learnt and grown considerably more than if I had not had my share of challenges; and have developed some level of empathy for my fellow human beings as we share this rich life journey.

Under the guise of the business of health, I am surreptitiously a health and life coach; and, though I attempt to 'walk the talk' as much as I can, I do not necessarily enjoy anyone observing me in my fragile and vulnerable moments. However, those moments have manifested more often than I would have liked, and sometimes very publically. Just when you think the mask is firmly in place for all to not see the real and human you, something triggers that part that *is* real and begs to be expressed. Out of left field. Just like that.

One such time was when I was at yet another workshop (No. 2340, I think!), when life conspired to co-ordinate a series of events to trigger some deep emotional pain in me. When that tender spot was finally triggered there was no stopping that swell of emotion that had been suppressed under that mask for far too long. The ice broke under a torrent of tears. Very uncomfortable for a good little perfectionist like me! Nowhere to hide! And this was not one of those touchy-feely workshops with group hugs and tissues-a-plenty, but one on finances and business management! Despite this, I felt the softening in myself, and those around me, as I was met with compassion and understanding.

Mask askew, make-up smeared, snotty nosed and blotchy, I realised others responded much more warmly to this version of me. It was very imperfect but very real.

For a number of reasons that workshop brought up much of my abundance and unworthiness issues. It was a very painful experience, but also a turning point in that it made me address the beliefs and thought-patterns I had long been ignoring despite experiencing their unhappy effects. Within the intense feeling of that emotional pain began the process of its dissipation. It was a lot less of an issue after my consciousness knew it had got my attention.

Life has a way of cracking open that protective shell, despite our fraught attempts to hold it together, when it no longer serves who we are becoming. We might call it a 'nervous breakdown', or even a 'dark night of the soul'; and Prozac is not necessarily the answer to those stirrings in your soul. Life has a way of triggering what needs to be *felt*, though we might fight tooth and nail to resist it. This is what crisis is all about. It will force us to address and change what we have previously ignored. We will get louder and louder signals until we take note, and these signals definitely include illness.

Of course it is best to not wait for a crisis to happen if we can avoid it. There are much more elegant and conscious ways to go about it. The more awareness of ourselves we have on a day-to-day, or even a moment-to-moment basis, the less we will have to experience crises, wake-up-calls or significant upheavals. Non-judgemental awareness of the ebb and flow of what we feel and insight into our underlying beliefs, which can then be matched with healthy adjustments, is the key.

In addition to being aware of what we feel, as best we can, on a moment-to-moment basis, daily review of our emotional reactions is a helpful practise. It helps to regularly sit ourselves down and have a good hard look at ourselves. This includes scanning our emotional reactions to what we have experienced, as well as our resultant behaviours and possible effect on others.

Of course meditation is a powerful method to get to know yourself. During meditation you use an aspect of your consciousness that can observe those parts that might be more awry. Meditation, and even contemplation, is a good way to practise being present with yourself on a daily basis. It is a means of becoming truly *conscious*, and averting the unconscious invitation to more dramatic ways of becoming aware of your mind/emotion content.

It is to your benefit to become non-judgementally aware of your feelings and emotions as best you can, gain insight as to why they are there, and then change them for the better. This is the process of maturing and transmuting them to a healthier form. This is indeed a work in progress and the road to wisdom. This is, in fact, a life journey.

Awareness versus 'Acting Out'

Many will be concerned that if we are honest with what we feel, we might be unleashing emotions that can potentially cause harm to self and others. There is a difference between having awareness of our true emotions, and acting them out. Feeling and expressing emotions is not about histrionic expression as that is itself a distortion which is, in fact, much more likely to occur when there is little emotional awareness, little awareness of self.

We are much more likely to act out our emotions, and often in very insidious and harmful ways, if we are not conscious of them. To add to this, whatever we express, especially if this is done *unconsciously*, might well trigger another's unresolved issues and tender points. This can give rise to the classic heated argument where wounded ego is fighting against wounded ego. If we do not have an awareness of what we feel, and why we feel it, we are also much more likely to project our emotional issues onto others and the world in general, and indulge in victimhood and blame.

I draw the distinction between pure emotions and 'mind generated' emotions. The latter is when the person is holding onto a *story*, which they are embellishing and perpetuating with exaggerated emotions. Pure emotions are honest. They are neither right nor wrong. They just are. Our minds will work overtime and attempt to rationalise what we cannot allow ourselves to feel. The less we feel, the more we think; and as is said, 'the mind is a great servant but a terrible master'. It is the thinking mind that can get us into all sorts of trouble yet be our greatest ally if working in harmony our heart – i.e. what we *truly* feel.

When we have not assimilated an experience and resolved the related emotions, we have a way of repeating the experience and reactivating these latent emotions. The classic example is unwittingly choosing a partner who has aspects similar to those of a parent with whom we might have unresolved issues. This is our unconscious way of trying to win the situation that we believe we had lost in our early life. This is a *no-win* situation for all involved, and cannot be resolved until we become aware of and change this pattern.

If we have a strong emotional reaction that is out of proportion to a current situation, very likely something unresolved from our past is being triggered. This is nature's way of bringing our attention to and resolving the original hurt – helped if we allow those emotions to be felt while maintaining some awareness of the process. If we think of a past situation and experience a strong emotional charge, this indicates that the issue has not yet been fully resolved and integrated.

Childhood Origins

Young children are often trained away from what they really feel. They might be taught that anger is wrong and therefore *they* are wrong for having anger, rather than exploring *why* they might be reacting in anger and then upgrading their understandings about life. Often just *allowing* the emotions of young children, if no harm is being inflicted, will help them to naturally mature, particularly if wise presence and guidance is employed. Emotions have a natural maturation process, and if we skip that part in childhood we might have to complete the process in adulthood.

When, in our formative years, we are taught that some of our emotions are wrong, shame will often overshadow what we feel. Shame very much adds to the pain as it goes to the core of our rejection and survival fears. Thus starts the process of suppression/repression and adapting to how we think others want us to be. We then learn to not read and trust our own emotional cues – our own guidance system. This removes us from who we naturally are and from our innate knowing.

When we are programmed to adapt to how we think society wants us to be, rather than listen to our own knowing and intuition, we will be off-track from our own genuine needs, wants and purpose. And particularly, we might well forget our inherent self-worth – our worth for just *being*, not just for achieving. This will set the scene for our over-adaption and trying to be whom we think significant others want us to be. Thus we apply the mask (often *perfectionism*) that fools nobody more than ourselves.

At an ego level we are trying to survive, to keep ourselves on the planet. That is a good thing as otherwise it would be too easy to leave if we are having a bad day, and that would not serve our growth and evolvement very well. To survive, we know we are largely dependent on the society in which we live, and particularly on our early caregivers. Thus most of us will adapt to those around us, at least to some extent. Of course this depends to a large degree on our relationship with our caregivers, and their skills as guardians.

We also fear being punished for expressing what we *really* feel, particularly if those emotions are judged as negative. This can give rise to a long-term habit of self-punishment as a trade-off for being punished by others, and as a way of appeasing those to whom we have handed our power. This is a deeply unconscious process.

Due to how the brain works, when we are very young all experience is directly absorbed without any cognitive interpretation or rationalisation. There is no intellectual context to pass those experiences by, so we absorb them directly and literally. All impressions are directly absorbed by our biological systems, which then adapt accordingly. The emotional/limbic parts of the brain are imprinted, and this has a powerful effect on our future emotional reactions to life situations.

An individual's nervous and endocrine system is being formed and organised in a climate of adaptation to the environment – physical and emotional – in which they have found themselves. This is also influenced by ancestral and genetic tendencies as well as one's individual predispositions. The aim of this adaptation is for survival. Biologically speaking, one has a better chance of survival if the physiological systems are geared to cope with that individual's particular environment.

The foetus is particularly sensitive to the environment of the mother as that is the environment into which it is going to be born and to which it has to adapt. Usually, the mother *is* the environment (or the main part of the environment) in those very early formative weeks, months and years. Our genetic predispositions are to adapt to the environment of our forebears as likely this is the environment into which we will be born.

What is experienced in the early, formative years is adopted as the norm, and even the 'comfort zone', by an individual's system. From the situation into which one is born and which is experienced in their early, formative years, one either develops the belief that the world is a safe place and they are safe in it, or the world is not a safe place and they need to be on guard and have defences in place to survive it. This sets the scene for the functioning of their physiological processes (on guard or relaxed) and their mental propensities. This becomes one's 'programming'. Of course this whole process is subject to numerous other factors, including what one brings with them into this life.

'So this is how the world is and this is who I am in it.' 'I am loved and nurtured and can freely and safely express who I am'; or, maybe, 'I am wrong as I am, have to hide who I am, and have to try to make myself *right* to be accepted by the tribe, in order to have my basic needs met (i.e. survive); or I have to be a radical rebel to survive this situation.'

Adverse life experiences, particularly when experienced in the formative years, can significantly contribute to one's separation from their authentic self and corrode one's trust in life. If one was not born into a 'feathered nest' and did not experience that love and nurturing that was their birth right, they innately knew that something was missing and would often spend their whole lives looking for it – often in distorted and destructive ways. On the surface they did not even know what was missing, but the deeper level of their being certainly did.

If one's early-life needs were not met in a healthy way this might have been perceived as the normal state that one would thereafter expect and attract. There might be no reference for experiencing otherwise. It might not even have been particular experiences but rather the pervading background emotional tone of their environment that caused the most harm. We well know that emotional *neglect* can cause as much harm as specific adverse experiences. Despite pain being experienced as the norm, and something one adapts to, there will be a deep discord related to this sort of existence.

It can be said that one's natural pure state was violated by certain experiences, and certain messages received, but more so by the conclusions one drew and perpetuated in response to those experiences. These give rise to the 'distortions' that can reside at a deep level of consciousness. Though we have our own individual predispositions, these distortions can be perpetuated down through the generations and horizontally throughout the community like wildfire.

The damage we carry forth from adverse early-life experiences is the falsity we have taken on about ourselves and our conclusions about other people and life in general. There really is no past. The problem is what we have carried and reinforced in the *now*, from previous experiences. Paradoxically, it is the misaligned defences and adaptations we have developed in our attempt to survive life that potentially cause the most harm to our biological and psychological systems.

An individual is formulating their own self-concept in response to what they experience, the messages they receive, the perceptions they develop, and particularly their conclusions about life. Some individuals are naturally more resilient than others and we know that different individuals are not necessarily affected the same way by the same circumstances. However, certain patterns prevail. Rather than the experiences per se, it is one's conclusions about life, their beliefs and related defences that cause the ongoing damage to their health and wellbeing.

When we have decided that we are just not good enough as we are, we will try to find ways to correct this. As previously said, we might over-adapt to how we think others want us to be. In this adaptation process we, unconsciously, decide that we need more or less of certain qualities to earn our keep on the planet, so to speak. As our body is a downward projection of what we hold in mind, it will also adjust accordingly, as these qualities have organ and physiological correlates. This can go down to a cellular level, and very specifically.

We might be conditioned to believe that we have to behave a certain way, live a certain life and *be* a certain way to keep our place in society. Many will harmonise society's demands with how they themselves want to live, very well. Others will not and will further remove themselves from whom they really are in an attempt to adapt and be accepted, and suffer a significant incoherence within their system. Awareness of this discord might well be further suppressed by society's approved-of addictions, such as alcohol, watching television, over-eating, gaming, etc. – much of which is just considered our normal way of life.

As the ego's job is to survive it will fight against or resist anything it feels will counter its survival tactics. Our conscious mind might recognise a habit that does not serve it well, but our more immature subconscious and ego mind will often not want to give up what it sees as maintaining its survival. After all we have kind of survived with these habits up to this point. However, if we remove ourselves from our distracting addictions, and really tune in, we will realise that the life we have created for ourselves has much room for improvement.

Furthermore, we can, paradoxically, become very much attached to those aspects of ourselves that we consciously do not like, recognise as destructive, and want to change – it is who we think we are at some level. It is familiar. We might, at an unconscious level, fear annihilation of ourselves if we get rid of those aspects that we have *unconsciously* identified with. Who would we be then?

It is a sure bet that if a lot of emotional pain is being repeatedly experienced, there is a wounded child lurking somewhere behind the adult façade. That child within us might still be seeking its unmet childhood needs, which, as an adult, cannot happen as the child would have wanted. When, as an adult, we become aware of this, we can alter the whole process. It is a matter of the mature adult-self being aware of and, with compassion, guiding that immature, wounded self. The *adult* has to be in charge.

Like the kindly but firm parent, it is best to deal with those aspects of our consciousness with understanding and compassion, rather than force. The task is to become more aligned with those higher aspects of our consciousness that can observe and entrain those more immature aspects. It is best to reclaim and transform that energy that has been tied up in those lower states, rather than have one part of ourselves fighting against another part. That is why *forcing* change does not work as it is one aspect of ourselves bullying another aspect, which just promotes further disintegration.

I do believe that some individuals *chose* more difficult early experiences to accelerate their growth then share their learning with others. I believe some chose to be those canaries that are more sensitive to the ills of society. Rather than being armoured with defences they allow themselves to feel. Society does not necessarily want to acknowledge, nor examine, its own shadow. Individuals, and the human society as a whole, need to *recognise* what is not serving them and from there evolve to what brings about greater health, wellbeing and mastery for all.

This discussion is not to *blame* parents, society and so on, but to recognise harmful patterns that clearly need to be acknowledged and changed. The messages we receive and the beliefs we formulate as children are crucial regarding later emotional and physical health. Prevention is better than cure. This is a societal issue, on one hand deeply personal yet part of what our society and the human species experiences as a whole.

No-one is perfect, nor had perfect upbringings and we *all* have some wounding. I do not think we would be here, on planet Earth, if we did not have something to work on and grow through. It is what we do with the hand we were dealt that counts.

I do need to acknowledge that overcoming some significant adverse childhood, and even later-life experiences and the messages and beliefs that were construed from these experiences, can be an enormous struggle and a lifetime journey for some. If there was significant trauma experienced at a very early age, emotions experienced in later life might be very chaotic, confused and difficult to decipher. If significant trauma was experienced this has to be healed. Appropriate care from professionals skilled in this area is often needed.

People who *were* born into a feathered nest, and who were fortunate enough to have their early needs such as love and nurturance met, might never fully understand those who did not. It might be a case of 'we don't get you and you don't get us, and don't even try.'

I have heard many spiritual teachers and personal development coaches suggest people 'just get over it' (or messages to that effect). Of course that *is* the ultimate aim; however, there might not even be a conscious memory to 'get over'. I suggest that if they have not themselves walked the same 1000 miles in those moccasins, they are simply not qualified to give advice – or judge. I suggest that if you have had these experiences, it is best to take advice from those who have successfully taken themselves through a similar journey.

Ancestral/Genetic Influences

In the medical context, we hear so often that a condition is due to 'genetics'. End of story. No question. This statement implies that genes are static and that if there is a genetic cause or influence on a condition we are the passive recipients and cannot do anything about it. We now know that genes are not static. It has been well established, through the study of *epigenetics,* that genes are but blueprints and their expression is subject to a multitude of factors, including (and maybe particularly) what we hold in mind.

We generally believe that our genes cause our thinking and psychological predispositions; however, we now understand it is also the other way around – that the way that we think affects the expression of our genes. And why would nature get it so wrong? Why do we passively accept that all of the afflictions and disorders we experience are due to a basic design fault in our genetic machinery? There has to be a bigger picture.

The biological imperative of the 'tribe' is to survive life on planet Earth. This includes survival of the descendants so as to propagate the species. At a purely biological level, nature is more interested in survival of the species than survival of the individual. Therefore our genes will reflect our biology's attempts to pass down survival advantages to ensure survival of the tribe. If something is unhealed, unresolved and unintegrated within the tribe, this will translate into a biological or psychological adaptation that is transmitted down the genetic line – to ensure its survival.

We tend to focus on the physical aspects; however, emotional factors have a significant impact on our biological adaptations. Nature or nurture? I would say both, inextricably interconnected, as is mind with body. It has now been demonstrated that information related to trauma and stressful events can be passed down the genetic line. Thus it appears that emotional memory – and biological correlates – related to the experiences of the forebears, are transmitted to the descendants. This makes sense from a 'survival of the species' perspective.

It appears that the emotional charge and the resultant adaptations (to avoid that emotion!) particularly have an impact on our genes, and thus biology. So the offspring might be compensating, *biologically*, for what was unresolved *emotionally* in the forebears. Genes, as blueprints, carry these adaptations; and the expression of the genes might be triggered given the descendant's circumstances, environment, mental characteristics and various other factors. So what is unresolved emotionally will have *biological*, as well as psychological and behavioural correlates or adaptations that will be transmitted vertically down the ancestral line.

We are obviously very connected to our genetic line but often do not recognise how profoundly this can affect us. We will, at some level, carry forth the unresolved issues of our forebears. The advantage of this is that what was not resolved and integrated in one generation has the opportunity to be so in later generations. We unwittingly carry forth our ancestors' issues so that we have an opportunity to heal them.

Though we are individuals, our experiences, lives and destinies are intertwined with those of others. We are not operating in this world alone. We are subject to myriad factors, including what we have inherited, biologically and psychologically, from our ancestors. Some of the issues an individual might be experiencing might be related to those they have 'taken on' from an ancestor. They might be unwittingly carrying forth an issue from an ancestor who they might not even have known existed, and this can have a profound influence on their way of being in the world.

I have seen a number of individuals where it is evident they, at some level, have decided that 'the buck stops here' regarding an issue that has been passed down their family line. These individuals deal with the issue head-on, becoming *conscious* of it, so that it does not continue to be *unconsciously* passed on through the generations. The issue will play out in their emotions and life, they will allow themselves to fully feel it rather than suppress it, and then seek ways to heal it. This will benefit their descendants and the community at large. Alternatively, it will play out in their bodies as illness and be further transmitted down the genetic line.

We do not live in a vacuum. Even though the modus operandi of life on Earth is that we live from our own individuality, we are inevitably, and often unconsciously – vertically and horizontally – affecting others in one way or another. We will teach and learn through our emotions and behaviours, positive and negative. 'The good, the bad and the ugly' – it is all part of the mix from which we learn and grow.

Acceptance versus Resistance

Acceptance of where we are at and what we are experiencing soothes any emotional pain. Awareness and acceptance go hand-in-hand and are the antithesis to resistance. When we let go of resistance and drop into acceptance there is an immediate relief of tension and we can then regroup to more calmly proceed with our lives. This does not mean we resign ourselves to unwanted circumstances, or 'give up', or maintain unhealthy emotions. It means that we accept the *now* circumstances, with all of its inherent lessons, from which we decide to create a happier outcome for ourselves.

The paradox is that the point of change is when we accept what is. Resistance will always maintain what we are resisting. When we allow 'negative' emotions to be genuinely felt they will naturally change and be replaced by much warmer, more pleasant emotions as the integration process unfolds. If they do not change then *thought* – holding onto the story and remaining in victimhood – is often still in the way.

Emotional release is about fully engaging and then releasing the energy of the unwanted emotion so as to create room for the wanted. The aim is to ascend the emotional scale. It helps to be discerning regarding with whom one expresses their emotions. Negative and immature emotions *can* be very destructive, particularly if let loose without any discipline. Of course one's negative emotions need to be managed. As previously noted, when there is little awareness of one's emotional content it is more likely to be expressed in an unhealthy manner; or be internalised to cause disharmony to one's physiological processes.

It is very different to express emotions in a context of healing and support – where the aim is to bring about emotional maturity and resolve the underlying misperceptions about life – than to express them in an atmosphere of rebuke and judgement. Supporting one in their emotional expression is not about drama, indulgence or pity; it is about shifting the emotions and the related misunderstandings and misconceptions about life. Compassion rather than pity should be employed. Compassion and pity are worlds apart. Compassion is a love-generated emotion with the overall aim of being solution-orientated, whereas pity is steeped in victimhood and hopelessness.

It should be noted that some people might have deep psychic wounds that can be very difficult to access. The deeper aspects of their being need to be reached to bring about effective change, and this might well require the involvement of practitioners skilled in this area. The subconscious sometimes needs to be treated with appropriate tools that can access it.

Particularly if an individual has significant psychopathology they will need the assistance of appropriately-trained professional practitioners to stabilise and treat them for the safety of themselves and others.

The bringing up of emotions should never be forced by a practitioner or client but rather, *allowed*. Forcing emotions has a falsity and can be re-traumatising and harmful. We have bunkered down those emotions for a reason and subconsciously we think we are keeping ourselves safe by not feeling them. I believe they will be triggered when and if it is the right time for them to be triggered, and our being knows when that time is. We cannot and should not force it as that, itself, is a form of self-rejection.

I have had many patients come into my consulting room who collapse into a flood of tears as soon as they sit down. The pent-up emotions finally have an opportunity to release, though the person often tries hard to gain composure, somehow seeing their honest emotional expression as wrong or shameful. We have been so trained to see emotional release as a failure! I am always relieved when the floodgates are opened as they have reached what is really disturbing them and are courageous enough to face it.

I have had patients enter my consulting room clearly seething with anger, and other emotions, yet seemingly unaware of this. They are often very demanding and often much focussed on their physical symptoms. As said elsewhere, over-focus on our physicality can be a great distraction from what is going on emotionally and mentally, which is usually where the core of the problem resides.

Such people can be like tightly-coiled springs about to release. They might remain fixated on tests and test results while ignoring their own inner dimensions of feelings. Sometimes it is difficult to point out to people that, regarding health and wellbeing, maybe reaching and resolving their deeply-buried pain might relieve their current tension and be the best thing for their overall health.

I am much more concerned when I know someone is suppressing the emotions as the tension is palpable and I have a sense of what it is doing to their bodies. It is very easy to get distracted by dealing with the surface stuff in these situations. I am also aware when the 'story', and particularly when feelings of victimisation, are exaggerating the emotions. The story can be a great distraction from one's true feelings. I know how emotional suppression feels in my own body and I am very grateful for those who have held the space for me while I have been able to feel and express my own emotions and sort out the related misconceptions I might have been holding.

Emotions as Guides

The variety of experiences that life subjects you to, allows you to recognise what you do and do not want to experience thereafter. You are in fact responding to your own created reality, which is dependent upon your thought-patterns, beliefs and attitudes. If you have supressed those emotions, and thus not *felt* them, they cannot guide you. If you put your hand on the hot stove, but could not feel the pain, you would not be aware of the ongoing damage your hand was being subjected to.

The process is about learning from all of your experiences and honing your wisdom to better understand how life works so as to better manoeuvre through it. This is an internal job. It is not about changing the external world but primarily about changing your internal world, including your perception of events and your point of attraction to all that you experience. When you change your perception, you change your experience of reality, which can be but a reflection of what you hold in mind.

Emotions are designed to come and go and inform us of the *vibration* of the related thought-patterns we are holding in our minds. If we have a positive thought that is aligned with how life works, and who we really are, we will feel good. If we have a negative thought – meaning not aligned with the truth of who we are and how life really is – we will feel bad. So emotions, through sensations in our bodies, will inform us of whether our thoughts are on track or not.

As previously mentioned, there are no rights or wrongs, even though we might label emotions as 'positive' or 'negative'. These are only descriptive terms and *all* emotions are useful in the information they give us. If we tune in we are informed and can adjust accordingly. If we suppress feelings and emotions we will not be informed and the underlying misalignment of thought will be perpetuated. Then we will get the message in another way.

If we do not like the reality we have painted and perpetuated for ourselves we will get emotional signals that indicate some change might be for our benefit. When we have awareness of these emotions, and the related thought-patterns, we are better able to adjust them to what better serves us. Life will always be guiding us in the right direction, so we do not have to force the issue. It can, and is best to be, a gentle, flowing process. It is about tuning in, moment-to-moment, as best we can.

Our emotional indications help guide us through life. We need to be able to *feel* the spectrum of emotions to have that reliable guidance. If we have decided we should not feel so-called 'negative' emotions such as anger or sadness, and we therefore suppress them, we will have an unreliable guidance system. Negative emotions are indicating that something is askew, including our underlying beliefs, attitudes, and perceptions, or general view of life. They might also indicate when something needs to be addressed or changed in our lives, such as an unhealthy environment or how we let ourselves be treated by others.

Our intuitive powers will also be hindered if we have neglected emotional growth and discouraged ourselves from the world of feeling. If we, in our early life, experienced some adverse experiences that corroded our trust, in later life we are much less likely to trust life in general and our own inner voice. Not trusting life equates to not trusting one's own intuition and connection to that higher universal intelligence. When we suppress emotions, and are unaware of our related beliefs and thoughts, we also suppress the whisperings of our own heart.

'Heart' will connect us with actual reality, free from the mind's misinterpretations. Heart and mind are meant to work together, with heart on lead. The heart knows and the mind is designed to implement that knowing. Heart, or intuition, is our connection to our true, inner self and to that universal intelligence. The heart knows to be in and to spontaneously *respond* to the moment, rather than *react* with habituated, learnt patterns of thought and behaviour. If the mind is untethered to the heart it will rationalise away from this innate knowing. The mind can be very clever in its justifications that keep us bound to our familiar, programmed way of being.

What has all this got to do with Physical Health?

You might well ask: 'What has all of this got to do with health and health care?' Mind and body work together and are different levels of manifestation of our one human system. I believe that far more damage is done to our bodies by these unrecognised, suppressed, unexpressed emotions, and related misconceptions about life, than by any external factor. In fact, one could say that the external factors are but a reflection of what we hold in mind, as our beliefs so affect our experience of life.

Regarding health, our thought-patterns and beliefs have a very literal, direct effect on our bodies. This is the power of the mind that we often overlook. The point of being aware of our emotions is to become aware of the underlying thought-patterns, attitudes and beliefs that often reside at an unconscious level of mind and that can directly affect our bodies. From a physical perspective, the body will respond to our mind-content in like. This is, of course, a deeply unconscious process.

Emotions are the interface between mind and body. Emotions are visceral and felt in the body. They are the body's translation of thought, particularly the *energy vibration* of thought. When we do not fully feel, and sometimes express and release our emotions, they remain in a suppressed or repressed form and reinforce the underlying belief patterns that help give rise to them in the first place. This affects the health of our bodies because our mind-content contributes significantly, and specifically, to the functioning of our physiological processes. Our bodies directly follow our thoughts and beliefs, most of which we are not consciously aware.

Think of one moment of anger or bliss, and note how quickly the body responds to these emotions. We are so familiar with these automatic body reactions to thought and related emotions that we become completely unaware of them. Transient thoughts and emotions are not the problem as they are designed to come and go – to flow. It is the *entrenched* thought-patterns and beliefs that are tied in with our unresolved experiences and issues about life, and which our suppressed emotions hold in place – that are the problem.

The body is continually interpreting and adapting to what we hold in mind. For example, if our underlying belief is that the world is not a safe place and we have to be on guard to survive it, this will affect the working of our autonomic nervous system, pushing it into a defensive, vigilant state. This of course will have an adverse effect on the body in the long term.

I see again and again clusters of illnesses in those who have had adverse early-life experiences, which includes not having had their early needs for love and acceptance met. Very often these people have courageously and cognitively dealt with their past but the evidence is that they are still carrying their past in their bodies. Their bodies have tried to adapt to their experiences and derived beliefs in the best way they know how. It is actually a very innocent though somewhat distorted process, and we probably all do this to some extent.

For example, there is a strong correlation between some gastrointestinal conditions and unresolved, particularly early-life, traumas. We are becoming much more aware of the brain-gastrointestinal tract link. At a mind-body level, the gastrointestinal tract correlates with the processing of life experiences. If there have been difficult and unresolved early-life experiences, often emotions are chaotic and unintegrated, with the functioning of the gastrointestinal tract responding accordingly.

(By the term 'trauma' I am referring to any experience that causes significant physical or psychological impact and pain, and that remains unintegrated and therefore unresolved, and from which certain maladaptive programming and beliefs have been derived. We have all experienced this to some extent.)

When we resolve and integrate our experiences, gain the learning and wisdom from them, and firmly put our sights on a healthy future, we will promote the coherence and healthy functioning of our biological and psychological systems.

Conclusion

The big question in my mind is: do we *transform*, or do we *transcend* our negative, painful emotions? Do we just rise above them and align with higher emotional states? Or, do we wade through them at an experiential level to integrate and transform them? I do believe that it is matter of 'different courses for different horses', or different courses at different stages of our development and evolution. There is no singular approach that applies to all people, as we are manifold in our experiences and predilections.

There is no doubt that if one had absolute wisdom, and harmony within themselves and with life in general, they would experience less disturbing emotions. They would have more emotional equanimity and experience a generalised, elevated feeling state – regardless of external circumstances. Emotions would still come and go as that is part of the human condition; however, they would be more like temporary ripples rather than major disturbances.

Our personality – that face that we present to the world and who we think we are – is often made up of the aspects of ourselves that have been conditioned and programmed away from what is real. This is endemic. The personality that is experiencing the pain is not the real self. Healing is dispensing with, or rather, transforming or transcending the falsity. Paradoxically, this starts with compassionately accepting where we currently are; otherwise it is too tempting to put another false self, like a veneer, over our currently unhealed aspects.

If we cannot emotionally feel what is not working well in our society, our humanness, ourselves, we will never change it for the better. We will not learn how to evolve out of it. Of course that should be the aim of any difficult experience – not to wallow in it as we can so easily do, but to recognise what is not beneficial for us so as to change it for the better. We will be subject to 'contrast' for our growth; and the contrast will cause us to step up and evolve our minds beyond what attracted the contrast in the first place. We learn from everything and probably more from what we would not (consciously) choose to experience.

I know personally, if I had not experienced some emotional pain in my life it would not have put me on the path of searching for solutions. This has led me down various tracks, all of which have been very interesting and informative in their own ways, all for my growth and learning. Hopefully I can share the best of it. Many of us might never fully heal the wound, but learn and grow considerably in the process of trying – to the extent that the wound fades into insignificance.

Essentially healing is acknowledging the innate innocence that is hidden under the layers of disturbances that might reside in our consciousness. In that innocence lies our basic human need to be loved and connected. All disorders of mind, body and spirit are related to our often-distorted ways of trying to get those needs met. Understanding this and seeing our potential to rise above it is where genuine compassion resides.

True healing is about dispensing with the falsity that we have taken on, coming back to whom we really are, and living our life accordingly. It is about being responsible for our own lives. It is also about seeing *another's* potential of being able to work through, learn from, and rise above their issues – if they so choose.

When we are attempting to change aspects of ourselves we need to do it for ourselves, rather than aiming to get another's approval, as that is just suppression and shame coming through the back door – repeating those patterns we are trying to rid. Always tune into your own intuition regarding what is right for you. I say it would be a pretty boring place if we were all the same, and our learning would be halted pretty quickly if that were the case.

The aim of all healing is to create happier, healthier and more fulfilling lives for ourselves. This includes unfolding from our past and learning the wisdom so as to be at peace with ourselves and with all of life. We might have to clear a few road-blocks related to our early life experiences, and more so what we have concluded from them, that lie in the way of our creating a happier future. Of course we also build upon the good we have experienced. Some would say we can change our past, or certainly our perception of it, and this includes being aware of the great growth our experiences have stimulated. It is about restoring trust in the unfolding of life and our place in it.

End of Chapter Points

- *Thoughts and emotions are concurrent and just different expressions of the same energy.*

- *Emotions are the interface between mind and body, the translation of thought into body feelings.*

- *The very awareness, and sometimes expression and release of emotions, starts their integration and transmutation to a higher form.*

- *When we suppress or repress our emotions and feelings, we are blocking the life force, the natural flow of energies.*

- *Emotions will remain at the level at which they were formulated and suppressed or repressed, despite intellectual prowess and maturity in other areas.*

- *Whatever we are feeling is the truth of the moment, regardless of whether we like it or not.*

- *Emotions are our indicators of the vibration of our thoughts and beliefs. We cannot adjust and correct that of which we are unaware.*

- *When we do not tune into our own feelings and emotions, it is difficult to tune into those of others.*

- *Feeling our emotions can feel like annihilation to the ego, so there can be a great deal of resistance to this.*

- *When we dull the capacity to feel, we dull the capacity to feel all emotions, including joy, and accordingly dampen our intuition and creative abilities.*

- *Adverse life experiences, particularly when experienced in the formative years, can start the process of emotional suppression, which significantly contributes to one's separation from their true selves.*

- *It is our conclusions about life, our beliefs and our related defences that cause the ongoing damage to our health and wellbeing.*

- *Regarding health, our thought-patterns and beliefs have a very literal, direct effect on our bodies.*

- *It is a sure bet that if a lot of emotional pain is being repeatedly experienced, there is a wounded child lurking somewhere behind the adult façade.*

- *Unresolved emotional traumas in the ancestral line can be inherited in our genes and potentially contribute to physical conditions in the descendants.*

- *The paradox is that the point of change is when we accept what is. Resistance will always maintain what we are resisting.*

- *Life has a way of triggering what we need to feel, though we might fight tooth and nail to resist it.*

- *Emotions are part of our inner-guidance system. Our emotions, by how they feel, will help us to recognise what we do not want to experience so we can start the process of changing this to what we do want.*

- *Healing is to access the wisdom of one's own heart, and to bring our trust back to the process of life and, particularly, to ourselves.*

Chapter 2

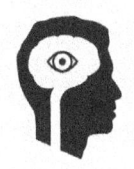

Consciousness: The Great Untapped Healing Tool

"Consciousness cannot be accounted for in physical terms for consciousness is fundamental. It cannot be accounted for in terms of anything else."

ERWIN SCHRODINGER
(1887-1961, AUSTRIAN, NOBEL PRIZE-WINNING PHYSICIST)

Evolving Understandings

We are living in very exciting times. We are at a time of profound and rapid transformation. Change is occurring rapidly at a global and individual level – have you noticed? We are at a time of changing paradigms and some of our old structures will not survive. We are de-programming some of the old programs that no longer serve us, that have proven to not be life and wellbeing enhancing. The positive potential of these changes is enormous. I am intrigued by how these changes might affect health care and contribute to the health, wellbeing and the personal empowerment of individuals.

We are currently rapidly expanding our understanding of the role *consciousness* plays in every aspect of our lives, including our health and wellbeing. This is having an impact on health-consumer demands and health-care practises. The 'holistic' model of health recognises that consciousness plays an integral role in health and illness. It recognises the influence of mind, body and spirit on our health and wellbeing; and that all are interdependent.

Quantum physicists and ancient mystics have come to the same conclusion that thought precedes form. This emerging understanding points to the power of our consciousness in affecting our reality, which includes the functioning of our bodies. This potentially will have profound effects on many aspects of our lives including health care.

Our real evolvement at this juncture is learning to harness the power of our own minds, rather than trying to control phenomena in the external reality. It is an internal job, with the perceptions of our outer reality being very much influenced by what we hold in mind. Some would cite that our outer reality is literally a projection of what we hold in mind. An analogy for this is our mind being a movie projector and our 'reality' being what is viewed on the movie screen.

Thought, which stems from brain, mind and consciousness, has great transformative and creative power, so it is to your advantage to use it wisely. Thought matched with emotion will set the vibration of what we attract into our individual and collective realities.

What is 'Consciousness'?

Consciousness is where it all happens. It is the bottom line of every other manifestation, including our bodies, our health and, in fact, our complete experience of reality.

By the term 'consciousness' I mean all that we hold in our mind at its many levels: conscious, subconscious and unconscious. We tend to equate the mind with the brain. I see the brain as the material and manifest working tool of the mind. The mind is also a product of the brain so they have a co-dependent, circular relationship, rather than a one-way linear relationship.

The brain translates what we hold in our mind into physical reality; and we know that the brain has enormous influence on the functioning of our bodies. We ground what we hold in mind into our body and actions through the brain. The brain puts into action what the mind designs. And where does the mind reside? Who knows? I don't see it as confined to the body.

For purposes of this exchange the word 'consciousness' is not used as in the conventional understanding of levels of alertness. I might use the words 'mind' and 'consciousness' interchangeably. I believe that consciousness is more expansive than, and encompasses, the mind. Consciousness is the all-pervasive energy that connects all phenomena.

We are also connected to, and influenced by, the 'collective consciousness', which includes our family, community, society, nation, and humanity in general. Dr David R. Hawkins, M.D., Ph.D. in his book *Power vs Force* states, "…the individual mind is like a computer terminal connected to a giant database. The database is human consciousness itself, of which our own consciousness is merely an individual expression, but with its roots in the common consciousness of all mankind."

Austrian psychoanalyst Sigmund Freud developed the concept of the 'unconscious' mind, though the term was coined earlier by 18th century German philosopher, Friedrich Schelling. The famous Swiss psychiatrist, Carl Jung, developed the concept of the 'collective unconscious.' These terms have now become common parlance.

Our individual and collective consciousness is connected to the field of energy, the overall consciousness that encompasses the all. Some might call this 'universal consciousness', 'source energy', 'life energy', 'chi', etc. The term 'universal consciousness' refers to the more expansive field of energy that is inclusive of every other field of energy and all phenomena. This is not a linear relationship, but rather a holographic relationship, where everything is connected to everything else and a part of the whole reflects the whole.

When referring to the effects of our consciousness on health we are referring to our individual consciousness/mind, but with the understanding that it is influenced by the collective consciousness and connected to the all-pervasive universal consciousness. Brain and body are the downward (yet concurrent and not separate) manifestation of consciousness.

Of course, we are interpreting these understandings through our limited intellects as best we can. Studies in quantum physics, and metaphysical studies, will give you a more in-depth understanding of this subject.

The 'Subconscious' Mind

My studies in kinesiology have given me more insight into the subconscious mind than has my conventional medical training. I am often amazed by what is held in our subconscious minds, and how it has such a strong influence on who we are and how we behave in this world. The subconscious mind has a lot to answer for! More on this subject later.

The terms 'unconscious' and 'subconscious' relate to what we hold in consciousness that is below our immediate waking awareness. 'Subconscious' refers to the mind-content that is just hovering below conscious awareness; whereas, 'unconscious' means the mind content that is far below our conscious awareness. For purposes of this exchange, I use the terms interchangeably.

Thought-patterns and beliefs can become so habitual they fade into the background of our mind (thus they are subconscious or unconscious), from which they still exert an enormous influence on the outworking of our lives. Of course we cannot be aware of all our unconscious mind content all of the time as it would be overwhelming to the conscious mind.

What we hold in our subconscious mind has a potent influence on our health, wellbeing and our experience of life in general. As previously mentioned, suppression of our emotions contributes significantly to the subconscious mind content that might adversely affect our health and wellbeing. Becoming *conscious,* or aware, of that which we have previously been *unconscious* of, is a significant part of any real healing.

The subconscious/unconscious mind is aligned with the workings of our bodies. Much of what happens at a physiological level is automatic, or 'autonomic', meaning functioning in the background below any conscious awareness. This is a necessary and efficient aspect of life, and works very well if our subconscious mind content is not awry. Candace Pert, in her book *Molecules of Emotion,* proposed that the body *is* the unconscious mind.

Dr Joe Dispenza, author of *Evolve Your Brain, Breaking the Habit of Being Yourself* and *You are the Placebo – Making Your Mind Matter,* has made enormous inroads into our understanding of the mind-body connection as it relates to brain, mind and consciousness; and has developed a methodology to enable us to change our subconscious 'habits'.

The efficiency of the mind-body has developed a method to tuck what has become automatic into the deeper recesses of our consciousness, where mind and body work as one. We have reinforced some of our thought-patterns so often that they take on an energy of their own and we do not have to exert any conscious effort to maintain them.

These thought-patterns so become our way of being that they are taken for granted, and therefore remain unacknowledged and unexamined. No problem if they serve us well; however, a significant problem if they do not. We have to take a step out of ourselves and have a good, hard look to see them; and we might well have to exert energy to overcome their habitualness. The life process alone will also continue to provide us with opportunities to upgrade our unconscious mind content.

If we have distortions in our beliefs and concepts regarding ourselves, and life in general, this will be held in the subconscious mind and will be reflected in our attitudes and behaviour – as well as in our physiology.

Regarding matters of health, we sometimes have our conscious mind and subconscious mind working in opposition. This will be discussed further in a later chapter. The task is to bring to light, without judgement, our subconscious mind content to see if it is working well for us or not.

This is the power of the *conscious* mind – to bring to awareness what has previously been hidden, so that one can examine its effects and adjust it for the better.

Consciousness and Modern Health Care

The practise of modern medicine is based on the Newtonian model of reality, which views matter – including our bodies – in mechanistic terms. The Newtonian model is based on the assumption that reality is made up of separate and independently existing parts. Separation of mind and body is still the dominant ideology in our culture and this is reflected in the practise of modern health care.

The modern belief in separation of mind and body had its origins in the 17th century. As the story goes, this was when Rene Descartes, the great philosopher, made an agreement with the then pope that if he was to use cadavers for scientific purposes, scientists would have nothing to do with the mind and soul. This dictate has perpetuated the belief that mind and body are separate, should be dealt with separately, and that only the scientific method is valid when assessing the functioning of the body.

It has also perpetuated the belief that because mind and spirit cannot be directly measured by scientific means, they are somehow less valid and less relevant, and are therefore often discounted in the world of health care.

Using the power of our minds to heal does not exclude other forms of therapy. I believe consciousness is inclusive of all and is infinite in its choices. When someone really decides to heal they will draw to them what is most efficient, what they are most aligned with, and what is in their best interests to bring about the healing. It might be very different for different individuals. It might be surgery or it might be an herb – or both. In our universe of infinite choices we really cannot judge what is best for any individual at any one time.

Do we Create our Reality?

People either believe there is a reality external to, and separate from, ourselves; or that all reality, at least to some degree, is a product, and projection, of our minds. The former belief is the conventional, agreed-upon belief, though it appears that this is now rapidly changing. These two different belief-systems give rise to two radically different ways of perceiving and operating in the world, and two radically different approaches to health care.

New understandings are enlightening us to the reality that our individual and collective consciousness affects our perceived external world. 'As within, so without.' This might not make a lot of sense to those who believe that reality is fixed and external to ourselves; and that is understandable because we have been so conditioned to see life this way.

Filtering into the collective consciousness at present is the ancient philosophy, and what many would believe to be a universal truth, that we create or co-create our reality. This involves the understanding that all we perceive and experience is a reflection, or a projection, of our consciousness.

It is the understanding that everything 'out there' is a mirror of, and determined by, our own thoughts, beliefs and attitudes – most of which are subconscious. We perceive reality through the filters of our own consciousness. We all have different views of reality as we all see life through different lenses, as determined by our individual life experiences, and our interpretation of those experiences.

To give an example: if we are both looking at a red apple we are unconsciously assuming that we are seeing the same thing and that the red apple is external to ourselves and has its own qualities independent from our gaze. We are both seeing the same red apple, separate from ourselves – obvious, right? That is the common, unspoken, unquestioned assumption for the majority of us.

However, when we examine this further, even using our 'common sense' thinking, we might understand that the retina at the back of my eye is not necessarily exactly the same as the retina at the back of yours; nor is my brain and its intricate connections and pathways exactly the same as yours. We perceive our agreed-upon, conventional reality through our five senses. So, we perceive the apple visually through photons hitting the retina at the back of the eye, triggering a number of neurological connections, which culminate in an image produced in the brain's visual cortex – of that red apple.

We will also *perceive* that apple in relation to our previous knowledge of, and experiences related to red apples. Our brains will sort out those connections. There might also be some emotional overlay that might influence our perception, depending upon our previous 'red apple' experiences. You and I perceive that apple through our own senses and neurological pathways as well as our previous experience and knowledge of red apples.

Obviously there is much commonality in all of this; however, it will not be exactly the same for every individual, despite our assumption that it is. It makes logical sense to me that there is no red apple that is completely independent of the perceiving consciousness. We *cannot* be seeing the same red apple. It is all smoke and mirrors. We are living in illusion.

Magicians create their illusions by taking advantage of the fact that we are continually predicting the next moment from our knowledge of the past. If we get enough clues we will 'see' what we are *expecting* to see. Paintings work the same way in that a few well-placed brush strokes will have the viewer create the rest, and even create a whole story in their minds – based on what they have experienced from their past.

Many metaphysical masters would say 'There is *nothing* out there that is separate from the perceiving consciousness; it is all a matter of perception.' You could say that we are all living an illusion of sorts; yet proponents of our conventional agreed-upon reality would say that to question the illusion – is the illusion, or delusion. When you do understand reality to be a reflection of what you hold in your consciousness, and all that that entails, you then know you can change the locus of control from outside to inside.

Though there is commonality and a shared reality to a point, we all perceive our realities through our individual brains, minds and consciousness. Two people can be in the same room but experience completely different levels of reality. The age-old question is: 'Does the mountain exist if there is no consciousness to perceive it?' Who knows? And, many would say: 'Who cares?'

And we might well say 'Who cares?' because it is easier to go along with our programmes and live life as we know it in our familiar trance state, rather than question reality and risk the disturbance. And it can be very disturbing and even crazy making to question our reality and our familiar lives; and, paradoxically, one has to be very well-grounded and well-guided to do so. However, be prepared for the ride of your life when, and if, you do question your programmed beliefs about the whole fabric of reality.

It can indeed feel very threatening to question our whole concept of how reality works; however, the potential for these understandings to revolutionise health care, and life in general, is enormous.

The Law of Attraction

The 'Law of Attraction' means that 'like attracts like' and that the situations we attract, and what we experience, are in direct relation to the vibration of our thoughts and related emotions.

Circumstances and experiences are matched and attracted to what we hold in consciousness, most of which is subconscious or unconscious.

This occurs no matter what age or state we are in. If we are not aware of the vibration we are emitting, we might well be confused and feel victimised by the circumstances we are experiencing. We might also be aghast and rejecting of the idea that we attract what we experience. This is not a punishment but rather for our growth in wisdom. It is life's way of giving us continual feedback on what we are putting out so we can adjust it for the better. It is a means of learning and evolving in this Earth-plane of existence.

I feel I need to issue a few words of warning on this subject. Firstly, most people on the planet, as far as I can see, do not yet have the understanding that they create, or co-create their own reality. In fact, that notion would seem preposterous, unscientific and even heretical to many.

Others believe that life will subject us to exactly what we need for our growth, with us being the passive recipients of life's lessons; that what we experience is not determined by us individually but rather there is a higher-life order at play that will provide us with exactly the experiences we need for our evolvement and the development of wisdom.

I believe both views are correct, but at different levels of our consciousness, with the latter being the *unconscious* model operating when we are still largely controlled by our unconscious programming. As we become more *conscious*, meaning more aligned with *universal consciousness*, and beyond our individual programming, we have more influence on the creation of our reality.

Secondly, we are currently living through exciting times where it appears that we *are* rapidly expanding our consciousness and learning to become masters of our own destiny. More and more people will understand that we are the main players in our own individual versions of reality; and it might well be our collective mission to undo the prior programming that suggests that we are not. We have been very well trained for a very long time to believe in an external reality that has nothing to do with the workings of our own mind. Many, I know, will be confronted by these ideas. I hope that changes – for everyone's sake.

I prefer to use the term 'co-create' as I draw comfort from the idea of a higher intelligence working with me behind the scenes. I believe that 'life' knows more than my individual ego version does and is reliably providing me with experiences for my growth. I would not like to leave the outcome of my life to my personality and ego alone! When mind and heart are working in unison, and we get beyond our subconscious programming, we are more likely to align with that higher intelligence, or however you might like to refer to it.

Thirdly, when we are still grappling with these understandings, it is very easy for shame to come through the back door, especially when we feel we have not yet become skilled at creating the life we think we want and are still experiencing suffering in one way or another. Our ego aims and wants might be very different to what our deeper being has called forth for its growth and development. Consciousness gets what consciousness needs for its expansion. Vision boards might not quite cover what is essential for our evolvement.

We can feel very disempowered when we have some understanding that we have a significant role in the playing out of our life, but don't yet feel we have the power to direct it as we would like. How we have been conditioned in early life has an enormous influence on this. I would suggest we let compassion and patience for ourselves, and others, trump shame. We have been trained in the opposite direction for a very, very long time. We are a work in progress and we always will be.

It is comforting to know that the circumstances we attract, which might trigger suffering, also serve to heal the glitches in our consciousness that attracted those circumstances in the first place. So life is always on our side if we allow it.

These concepts have a huge impact on understanding the mind-body connection and the follow-through implications regarding health care. As mentioned, the Newtonian model currently determines how we generally conduct health care. The Quantum model, which appreciates the primacy of consciousness, and questions our long-held understandings of the fabric of reality, might well turn health care on its head.

The Power of Thought

Mind/consciousness is the great untapped healing tool. Your greatest healing resource is your own mind. You can be very influenced, positively and negatively, by those around you, but nobody can control how you think – though they might try. Using our minds for healing does not preclude the utilisation of other health-care therapies/technologies; in fact, they can be used synergistically.

You might not have been taught how you can direct thought, and that this is a skill you can hone through practise. You might often be on auto-pilot, acting out of the habituated thought-patterns and beliefs you have developed, acquired or been conditioned to. It is for your benefit to take your power back, become aware of your thoughts and beliefs, and discern whether they are working well for you or not. This might involve healing the trauma that gave rise to them in the first place. This has enormous implications on your health and the very quality of your life.

Look around you. Everything that you see started with a thought. Everything that has been created started with a thought, often fuelled by inspiration. Buildings, cars, roads, clothes – all started with a thought. We habitually underestimate the power of thought, of mind. It goes way beyond creating 'things'. It creates your very reality, your whole experience of life – down to the finest detail.

Thoughts are like *things* in that they are made up of energy that can interact with the energy of anything else. We generally cannot see thoughts (though I am sure there are those with highly-tuned perceptive powers who can) so we consider them ethereal and not as important as solid matter, forgetting that they are interacting with matter in every moment. In fact, thoughts don't dissipate, as they are not subject to entropy like matter.

Ongoing and repetitive thoughts can become 'thought forms' and these have a more potent effect than passing thoughts. These thought forms then attract similar thoughts that will compound and maintain the theme. Agreed-upon thoughts and concepts create shared realities that we might, as a group or collective, buy into and further energise into reality.

'Reality' is responding to thought in every moment, so best to have good awareness of what you are putting out there. This is not as arduous as it sounds and becomes easier with practise, and is indeed a work in progress. One does not have to lose spontaneity in the process; however, impulsiveness and reactivity might become less.

As everything is connected, what we *individually* think will affect the all. Moment to moment. That is a very sobering thought. However, there is a balance between being aware of our thoughts, without judgement and while maintaining some spontaneity, and not being over-zealous in having to maintain positive thinking. Positive thinking can be a veneer that covers unexamined mind-content. Awareness is key. Better to be aware of something that is not working for you than have it buried and unexamined.

Particularly, the working of our bodies is constantly responding to our mind-content – most of which is subconscious. The body is a great indicator of what we hold in mind, as there is a direct feedback mechanism at play. This is not a punitive process – though it can feel like it at times – but an abeyance to the mind's dictates. This is why it is so important to 'know thyself' and get very acquainted with what you hold in your own mind. This includes thoughts, beliefs, attitudes and emotions.

We have to dispassionately assess ourselves from a higher level of consciousness, without judgement; in fact, with love, compassion and even humour. Maybe, particularly humour.

Intention

'Intention' refers to the deliberate directing of thought to bring about a desired outcome. It all starts with intention. Strong intention, aligned with powerful emotion, can move mountains.

Intent – positive or negative – is powered by strong emotion. The emotion fuels the thought to create *intent*. The strongest intent is matched with a knowing that what we intend is *definitely* going to happen, and projecting gratitude that it is already a done deal fortifies the process. This is a very different energy to wishful thinking, or hoping, underlying which is a subconscious but dominant concern that the desired outcome might well *not* happen. These energies feel very different in our bodies and this indicates how aligned (or not) we are with what we want and how much resistance is in the way.

At a deep level of our consciousness we can exercise negative or positive *intentionality*. Positive intentionality is pro-life, whereas negative intentionality is anti-life. Positive intentionality aligns with growth, wisdom, love, harmony and all that supports the best of life; negative intentionality aligns with all that blocks these qualities and is based on a fundamental lack of trust in life and all the good that it can provide.

These are very deeply-seated attitudes that are often the response to life experiences, and they will have a marked influence on the out-working of one's life, including one's health. These attitudes are well below conscious awareness and few people want to explore these hidden dimensions; and, in fact, ideally should only do so with expert guidance. However, intent is *intent*, regardless of the level of consciousness in which it resides, and bringing light to these areas will allow one the opportunity to change them. This is dealing with the shadow aspects of our consciousness.

With regard to health care, strong positive intent from patient and practitioner alike will help to bring about desired outcomes. Strong intent has a very different quality to taking the 'fighting' stance. Intent is harnessing the strong energy of thought and emotion in a coherent manner rather than opposing aspects fighting each other.

Many years ago, when my younger son was quite young, we were taking an interstate trip to Sydney for the weekend. This trip was very important to him as this would be his first time on an airplane, and we were all looking forward to a short break. My son was very excited to be going on his first plane trip and I was very much looking forward to sharing that experience with him.

As we were setting out I had a very uncomfortable feeling that we were running late and would not get to the airport in time to catch the flight. We also found ourselves in heavy peak-hour traffic, which further delayed our travel to the airport.

I expressed my dismay and looked around to see my son in the back seat of the car. He was trying to be very brave but I could see the disappointment on his little face. I could not bear to let him down. At that moment I declared to myself (and to the Universe!) that this was *not* happening, that somehow we would catch that flight and enjoy the weekend as planned. I remember the very strong determination I felt at that time – it *was* going to be! I did not know how, but it was going to be. I then looked again at the schedule and noticed the time of the flight had changed – we had an extra hour that would get us to the airport in time.

Had I read the schedule incorrectly in the first place? Maybe. Maybe not. And it does not matter because either way, the strong emotion I felt, married with my thoughts, brought about the results I had intended.

We have all heard stories of people who have performed feats that defy our beliefs of what is possible or not. We have heard of the mother who lifted a car off her trapped child, because in that moment her intention to save her child was much greater than any belief that suggested that this could not be done.

Regarding health care, the *intention to heal* has a very different potential outcome to that of maintaining the focus on the problem.

The Mind-Body Link

What has all this talk about consciousness got to do with our bodies and health?

I write from the premise that mind/consciousness and body are totally interdependent and work together. This just makes sense to me; and there is plenty of elegant scientific proof to verify these understandings for those who need it. What affects the mind will affect the body and vice versa. How could it not? The body is a manifestation, or downward causation, of what we hold in consciousness. There actually is no separation of mind, brain and body but we humans have tried to make sense of it all by designating separate parts. Consciousness encompasses and pervades it all.

It is still largely unrecognised that the mind has enormous power over the body – positive and negative. It is just that we have been programmed to believe otherwise. Clearly the mind is connected to the brain and the brain to the body. The body, with its physiological processes, chemical reactions and energy flows, is translating thought moment to moment.

Our health-care paradigm focuses primarily on external factors rather than on the workings of our consciousness. It focuses on what can get us and what we can be given to get over what can get us. We often treat our bodies as though they are completely dissociated from our minds, almost like a marionette that just gets us from point A to point B. Our thoughts are seen as less significant than what can affect us from outside of ourselves. What we hold in consciousness, what goes through our minds, is generally considered almost irrelevant, just background stuff. Well, that background stuff has a potent influence on your health, as well as on your life in general.

Some people become absolutely obsessed with avoiding perceived external factors. This might include being extreme with diet to the extent that many foods are seen as the enemy and a major threat to health if consumed. They might be particularly focussed on tests that check various biochemical factors and be overly concerned about numbers on paper. That all has its place and common sense does have to prevail; of course we need to treat, nourish and support the body appropriately.

However, many people appear to be completely unaware that certain attitudes or thoughts they are holding might be causing much more harm to their biological systems than the avoided external factors and details of certain biochemical reactions.

The body will let us know, one way or another, what we are holding in mind, and will often do so before the intellect does. It is particularly what we are harbouring in our *subconscious/unconscious* mind that is so reflected in the body as they work as one. What we hold in our minds can directly affect our bodies; and very specifically, pending the nuances of our thoughts and beliefs.

As the body is more aligned with the unconscious aspects of mind, one often has to reach these levels of mind to effectively bring about change. There are many methods available to access these deeper aspects of mind, including meditation, hypnosis and kinesiology. The aim is to bring what is in the subconscious/unconscious mind, where the programmes reside, to the light of *conscious awareness* – where choice can be exercised. Life will be doing this regardless.

Much of the body is operating at an autonomic level, and this is absolutely necessary to ensure our physical survival in this world. We *do* need to keep our heart beating 24/7. We *do* need our gastrointestinal tract digesting and processing our food without our awareness. If we need to defend ourselves or run away (fight or flight), the body does need to redistribute the blood circulation so that it can do what it needs to do in a flash.

The body knows what to do. It is when we do not believe this, and when thoughts and emotions are askew, that the natural processes and autonomic flow can be disturbed. The more unconscious these disturbed thoughts and related emotions are, the more they will affect the body. This does not mean that a passing negative thought or emotion will adversely affect our bodies – we would be in big trouble if that were the case. As previously mentioned, the problem is more the entrenched disturbed beliefs about life, which are often related to our unresolved and unhealed life experiences.

It is when we misinterpret life, and superimpose our judgements upon our human experience, that the body will react in kind. It is as though the body is trying to compensate for what the mind judges as amiss or incomplete in one's being or one's life. There is often a strong survival fear underlying this process. If we recognise and deal with our issues at the level of our minds and emotions – when we become *conscious* of them – the body will be less adversely affected. In fact, we will set it free.

We will develop physiological compensations for what we hold in mind. This can be very specific and literal, affecting certain aspects of the body that pertain to those aspects of mind. Why do we have such a plethora of illnesses and body conditions? Why do we not just suffer from an amorphous 'un-wellness' without any variation in symptoms and body manifestations? This reflects the complexity of our human system and our thought processes and life on this planet.

When we believe that life is on our side our bodies will more likely work in harmony. When we do not trust life or ourselves, this will be reflected in our mind and brain and then be translated into our bodies. Illness can be seen as being due to our not understanding and aligning with life's natural intelligence. Healing is to access the wisdom of one's own mind-body, where it is aligned with that natural intelligence, and to bring our trust back to the process of life and, particularly, to ourselves.

When you are attuned to and comfortable with yourself, as you are, and you experience life without judgement, your body will reflect that harmony. This does not mean that you do not change what you need and want to change, as this will be an ongoing process; rather that you are accepting of and true to who you are in the now. Paradoxically, that might include your wanting to change some aspects.

When you deny, judge, or reject yourself and strain to be something other, your body will respond with disharmony. There will be incoherence in the system. True healing is not about creating a false you. It is about coming home to your true self, to the core of who you are, and dispensing with, or transforming, the attitudes and beliefs that impede that.

Health is more likely to be the outcome when one is in harmony with who they are and with the flow of life.

"Show Me the Scientific Proof"

As Albert Einstein said, *"the significant problems that we have cannot be solved at the same level of thinking with which we created them."* If we are addressing something, scientific experiment or not, within a certain frame of reference such as prevailing belief-systems, we will not see possibilities beyond those predetermined beliefs.

It is *scientific* to think laterally beyond previously agreed-upon notions. Of course healthy discernment and scepticism is appropriate and necessary; but there is a large difference between that and emotional opposition to anything new. There is a difference between healthy scepticism and superstition. We did believe once that the world was flat! The notion that the world might be a sphere was seen as outrageous and heretical in its time, and pity those who chose to upset the status quo.

We are innocently gullible, and therefore easily programmed; and it suits some parties very well that we are so. Of course it is reasonable to stand back for a while and assess this new idea/concept/thing before jumping in boots and all. There is some crazy stuff out there and one indeed has to be discerning. However, that is very different to the emotional reaction of rebutting something because it does not support one's personal agenda or might put one out of their comfort zone.

In the medical world there is a compelling attachment of the collective ego to the scientific method. Anything seen as unscientific is often considered quackery, dangerous or suspect at best. Yes, of course science has a very big place; however, it should also be seen in perspective. If something is not scientifically proven and 'evidence-based' it is very suspect in the eyes of the medical world. Science has become the new God to whom we bow.

I am amused by the political correctness of being seen to uphold the scientific method. "Show me the studies, the scientific proof." "I am a man/woman of science." I hear this over and over in the medical world. It is like wanting to be seen as belonging to some superior intellectual society, where anything 'unscientific' is viewed as foolish nonsense.

We easily forget that the practise of medicine is as much an art as a science. We have invalidated and become distrustful of our inner knowing, simple logic, and intuition. Not to mention good old common sense.

When discussing various healing techniques, I have heard countless times – "Is it scientifically-based?" That is often rattled off without any real awareness of what is actually being asked. What exactly does 'scientifically-based' mean? Does it mean that if it is proven in a laboratory or by some form of statistical analysis it is credible? How does one prove an emotion or inner growth? That statement is also assuming all scientific experiments are 100% accurate, beyond any reproach and without any human bias or fallibility. We simply know that that is not the case.

If scientific endeavour is conducted within our already existing belief framework, we will be re-proving what we already believe. This is until we well and truly think outside the box. It is an inevitable part of our human nature that we will evolve our beliefs and understandings. Contradictorily, we are also universally threatened by change.

The common scientific method is based on the assumption that there is nothing beyond our perceptions, our five senses; and by corollary nothing exists beyond what we can observe and measure through these senses. This is quite limiting don't you think? It is like trying to look at the world from within a closed box with a pile of tools with which to look at phenomena within that closed box.

It is often more of a case of 'I will see it when I believe it', rather than 'I will believe it when I see it.' There is much resistance to new understandings that challenge the status quo of prevailing belief-systems. This is because it is perceived as a direct insult to the ego itself, as our beliefs are part of who we think we are. Most people do not want to risk the necessary change, this being particularly so if current beliefs and ways of doing things are tied up with one's perceived power and financial base.

People generally do not like change, even when what they are holding onto is not serving them well. This particularly applies to beliefs. We attach our egos and our survival to our beliefs; therefore, we can feel very threatened when these beliefs are questioned. This applies particularly when looking at something that so heavily impacts our lives as health care. Who would dare question current systems when they seem to be working satisfactorily? I beg the question – *are they?* We often choose to remain 'happy to be miserable' rather than risk change and upsetting familiar ways of doing things.

As a young doctor I did not question the system or what my superiors and the medical hierarchy dictated. It was only when I was taken out of that environment for a while and spent some time where I was presented with a different world-view that I started to have some questions. Life provided me with the opportunity to upgrade my beliefs. The new ideas (new to me) and concepts I was presented with just made sense and resonated deep within me. It was like coming home. I could see, in retrospect, that what I had earlier accepted did not fit with what I intuitively knew.

We assume our beliefs are logical and that anything that might threaten them is not. However, they are sometimes far more emotionally-based and visceral than logical. We attach logic to what we *believe* and to what is agreed upon by those with whom we feel we need to align. And we often feel that we need to align with certain groups for the survival of our reputation, credibility, power-base, income, if not our very existence. I have often seen this 'logic' displayed, knowing that emotional attachment to fixed ways of doing things is an underlying factor.

Humans evolved to introduce the scientific method as a way of growing beyond religious dogma and control; however, 'scientific proof' has become the new dogma and we can be as emotionally attached to it as we collectively were to the former. We have made 'science' beyond reproach, sacrosanct. Blind faith in science is actually an emotional response and very *unscientific*.

Everything that we believe is 'out there' is run through our perceiving consciousness, which will put its own interpretation on it. There is no purely objective reality. That is the illusion. We cannot isolate phenomena from what we perceive. All phenomena, in this reality, has to pass through our five senses, which will in turn be influenced by our own brains and the content of our own minds. There is always a subjective factor. That is logical.

It is generally accepted that everything has to be measured and dissected into smaller observable parts to be considered valid.

But not everything is *measurable* nor can be directly perceived through our five senses or by the means and techniques currently available to us. Consciousness does not care if it is proven and measured (good luck in trying!) or not. It will just keep on doing its thing regardless.

Can results of laboratory experiments and randomised trials be unquestionably translated into clinical practise? Do statistical analyses and agreed-upon consensus always push us in the right direction? I would think that history has proven otherwise. Ideally there is a balance between what can be gleaned from modern science and from time-proven empirical knowledge and experiential knowing. Though there is much commonality, no person, and no health issue experienced, will be exactly re-producible. There will always be a distinctive, individual flavour that cannot necessarily be measured.

In our culture we have developed the intellect at the expense of other more subtle, though powerful, aspects of human consciousness. We have also attached our collective egos to our intellectual prowess, and tend to invalidate other qualities such as intuition and the world of emotions. These other aspects of our consciousness are deemed more nebulous, more feminine, and somehow less relevant than intellectual aspects. We have given away our innate 'knowing' at the altar of hard scientific facts.

What is – *is*, regardless of proof. 'Lack of proof does not mean proof of lack.' Whatever we are measuring is now past tense as we are ever-evolving. We try to define and pin things down as though they are static and we can determine our future by them; however, they are ever-changing, slow it might seem at times. Science often tries to prove what is already there – past tense, not necessarily what is becoming. However, when science employs *creativity* and *inspiration* the outcome is often very beneficial, as we well know.

There will never be finite knowledge. There is no finite anything. Life just does not work that way. As we are ever-evolving, so too are the goal posts ever-moving. We will never dissect down to that last particle that holds all the answers. I have attended many medical meetings where professionals are grappling over minute details of specific biochemical pathways, looking for that special key. 'If only we could twig that particular pathway or adjust that chemical we could find the cure'. I wish it were that simple!

We are not machines. We are complex bio-energy systems, where all components are interconnected to act as a whole. Therefore we need to be treated as a whole. In health care we can so easily be obsessed with results of tests and data whilst overlooking the essential humanness of our patients. Patients can be particularly focussed on test results while forgetting their very selves.

On the other hand, scientific endeavour obviously has its brilliance and is a part of the evolution of our species. It enriches our world, enhances our understandings and adds to the ease and enjoyment of day-to-day life. Clearly in health care, many beneficial developments have come about – through science – that help enhance the health, wellbeing and lives of many. Of course we should take advantage of these wonderful developments. I am very thankful for them and enjoy them on a daily basis.

Scientific endeavour is expanding, as we are, and some brilliant and elegant research is being undertaken to look *beyond* what we have collectively agreed upon. There are some great scientists/ researchers who are currently conducting very innovative research to make more understandable and credible what they have been inspired to share for the benefit of humanity. When science is based on inquiry, creativity, curiosity and lateral-thinking it can be the means by which we humans apply the best of our intellects, and intuition, for the benefit of all.

The pendulum swings, as pendulums do. Ideally there is balance between the intellect and the intuitive aspects of our being. When one delves deeply enough, we understand that science and mysticism merge, as attested by some of the famous minds throughout the ages as well as those in current times. These people are philosophers and mystics as much as scientists, as they do not work on the premise these realms are separate.

Whose 'Scientific Proof' is Valid?

As was famously stated by Arthur Schopenhauer, *"All truth passes through three stages. First, it is ridiculed. Second, it is violently opposed. Third it is accepted as being self-evident."* The ridicule stage is when the perceived threat is small. The violent opposition phase is when there is a significantly large perceived threat.

In recent times, in my area, there was outrage from certain groups in response to some of the larger universities introducing some 'alternative' health-care courses into their faculties. Mainstream health care was not too concerned when these courses were taught in little colleges tucked away out of sight somewhere; but the fear and indignation rose in response to these prominent universities deciding to be inclusive of these courses. Now the threat is real. The ridicule has not worked. Those who only hold to the traditional, conventional paradigm of health care have indeed been threatened.

The big argument was that these health-care systems were not scientifically proven, that they should be evidence-based. In terms of health care, healing, and promoting wellbeing what exactly are we measuring and who decides what the correct 'evidence' is? In fact, who decides what 'healing' is and who has the right to dictate to another what healing is for them? Healing, indeed, is a very personal thing. No single group or system has *ownership* of health care; nor can precisely define what healing actually is.

Many complementary health-care courses *have* joined the world of 'evidence-based scientific proof', so those who are very suspicious of the world of snake oil should be happy their own standards are being applied. You can't have it both ways, guys – you either ridicule other health-care systems as being 'unscientific' or you embrace their entry into the bastion of intellect and science.

And why don't we look for the good before the bad? Why don't we actually open our eyes to see the benefit that many gain from holistic health care and natural therapies, in addition to that from conventional health care? Everything has its place.

We would all agree that the safety, protection and good care of the client is paramount, and it is clear that appropriate standards do need to be upheld. Same rules across the board, I say. We cannot overreact to a one in a million adverse reaction to an herb, whilst largely ignoring the much more commonly experienced side effects of many pharmaceuticals. It is often overlooked that iatrogenic causes of illness are alarmingly high.

Regardless of health-care discipline, there is the potential for the positive and the negative; and this comes down to individual practitioners in addition to the particular disciplines or methods practised. And no system, or individual, is perfect.

In the ideal world different health-care disciplines truly complement each other; each maintaining a high and safe standard and offering their own areas of expertise for the overall benefit of the health-care consumer; each acknowledging their own and the others' skills in an atmosphere of positive exchange, learning and respect. I look forward to a time when we have this integrative, cooperative, win-win system.

In the Name of Science

In any area of life, including the world of science, when mind and heart are working together, when intellect and intuition find a balance, the outcome is likely to be positive. When the heart is shut off in the name of 'science', the outcome can be dire – as history has proven.

On the front page of a recent newspaper was an article about a monkey farm, where primates are being bred for scientific experiments. The justification was that these experiments are *crucial* to bio-medicine and drug testing. I bet the monkeys do not think they are crucial. These animals are subject to unimaginable sufferings at the hands of people who are in the business of enhancing health and wellbeing for one species – ours.

Has anyone else noticed we are a very narcissistic, self-obsessed species? Who gives us the right? The pervading belief involved is that humans are superior and any other species can be sacrificed for the sake of our survival. We are conditioned to believe this, and we so unquestionably believe it that it remains unexamined and unstated by the majority.

How many people working in these areas, at all levels, would have to shut down their hearts and natural compassion to do this sort of work? I am certainly guilty of having, in the past, shut down my own heart for the sake of what was deemed necessary in the name of medicine or science. It is not just that the animals are sacrificed; it is the amount of suffering they are subjected to that is unconscionable. Try putting yourself in their position. Or your loved ones. The only argument that we can use is that we are more valuable than they are and that it is okay to do anything to another species for our sakes. And we have done this – human to human.

And what does 'crucial to bio-medicine and drug testing' really mean? It means we will go to any length to inch out a few more months or years in human-life expectancy. This is based on our distrust of our own bodies, and our unacceptance and fear of death. We think we can control death by external means, and will go to any length to do so. It is also so we do not have to suffer the inconvenience of an itchy rash or such, related to the use of cosmetics and similar substances; precious little things that we are.

It is also assumed the measured effects of various experiments on tortured laboratory animals that are living in a markedly unnatural environment, can be extrapolated to clinical practise. This is based on the flawed premise that there is a direct linear relationship between what is concluded from laboratory experiments on confined animals, and what will affect us humans as we are going about our day-to-day lives.

In some rat experiments that involve testing various substances for endurance, rats are left to swim in a tank from which they cannot climb out, until they surrender to exhaustion – to determine which substance gives the most staying power. Imagine for one minute how that would feel. Hearing of these things makes me want to scream in anguish and despair at our heartlessness. Conclusions from such research also ignores the multitude of factors that impinge upon how our minds and bodies function, assuming there is a simple linear relationship of cause and effect.

We largely hold the belief that the animal, plant and mineral kingdoms are at our disposal. Animals truly sacrifice themselves for we humans – much more than we realise. This does not just involve 'experiments' as mentioned above. They are teaching us and helping us all of the time – if we would just tune in. Animals are much more in harmony, instinctively and intuitively, with the natural world and the flows of life. I sincerely hope they will be viewed and valued much more than has been our tradition. Of course this goes for the plant and mineral kingdoms as well – and the Earth as a whole. We are just a part of it. Let's get over ourselves.

Tribal Bonding

No-one wants to stray from the group especially when they are deemed authorities and hold power. No-one wants to be seen as a maverick, or worse, a complete 'nutter'. No-one wants to be laughed at or dismissed and invalidated. No-one wants to be dragged away and labelled insane or even worse if they are not in agreement with those who hold power. This all taps into our deep survival fears. Being rejected from 'the tribe' is the number one fear for most us, even more than death. Well, it is a form of death as we are communal creatures.

Clearly many throughout history have been persecuted for thinking outside the square. These individuals had enormous courage and conviction in the face of enormous threat. They saw beyond collective agreed-upon beliefs and structures that did not serve humanity well; they stood for reform, no matter what.

'Rhino'

After graduating from medical school I spent four years training in city hospitals. One of those years involved doing a junior surgical residency rotation at a large hospital, where I was in the heart (or should I say *mind*) of medical patriarchy. Typically my workdays involved many hours assisting in the operating theatre, and many hours doing my ward work around my theatre time. Long and exhausting days to say the least! It was what was required and one of the many hoops junior doctors had to jump through to earn their kudos.

One of my hospital rotations involved working on the neurosurgical ward. The chief neurosurgeon was legendary for his toughness and dislike of women in medicine. Let's call him 'Rhino'. I have memories of having to call Rhino, often at night, when a neurosurgical case came through Accident and Emergency. He was not the most approachable person in the middle of the day, let alone when awoken from his slumber in the wee hours of the morning. His answers to my complex descriptions of a person's injuries or condition were usually met with monosyllabic grunts expressed with seething anger. His advice on how to manage seriously injured patients would go something like: "Broken leg, broken head – won't survive." Then he would slam the phone down, leaving me trembling and none the wiser about what was best for the patient.

As said, he clearly did not approve of women in medicine and particularly young ones with long hair. When he saw me on the wards he would often make derisive comments and then snigger with his sycophantic registrar as they walked off. Very challenging when I had to work on his ward for a number of months. It was then that I had the sting of knowing what being subject to prejudice was like. I realised there was absolutely nothing I could do to redeem myself as I had already been judged, and condemned, for who I was. It had nothing to do with my abilities, personal qualities nor potential, as they were just not seen.

Of course 'Rhino' was a brilliant and well-respected neurosurgeon. When you can open up people's skulls and operate on their brains you have enormous responsibility and wield enormous power. I actually have the highest respect for good surgeons – they are beyond courageous in going where the vast majority of people dare not. And, that experience for me those many years ago, was more 'grist for the mill' of life's way of toughening me up – somewhat; one of the initiations into the rigors of medical practise.

As a young doctor those many years ago, I did not question what the medical hierarchy dictated. When we are stretched and under pressure there is not a lot of room for lateral thinking or for questioning current systems and the powers that be. I would hardly be talking about mind-body medicine in the above setting. Suffice to say that to express an opinion that strays from that of conventional medicine, in some quarters, is fraught with danger.

Change filters in gradually until what was previously viewed as new, novel or even crazy concepts gets a hold in our collective consciousness and becomes the new normal. We do our individual bit in bringing about change but we cannot push the river. Maybe what we know, understand and are experiencing at any point, and the rate at which change comes about, is playing out perfectly.

Mystery

And where does 'mystery' fit in, dare I ask? As Max Planck (physicist, 1858-1947) stated, *"Science cannot solve the ultimate mystery of nature. And that is because, in the last analysis, we ourselves are... part of the mystery that we are trying to solve."*

Personally, I do like a bit of intrigue and secretly hope our human brains will not figure out exactly how life works. That would be a little mechanical, don't you think? It would be like ripping the curtain away from the wizard of Oz, to reveal something humdrum behind all the mystery and drama. Thankfully, I do not believe it will ever happen – not while we are in human form anyway. I suspect part of the game plan of life on Earth is to not fully know what the game plan is.

The intellect is but one aspect of our being and might never understand, nor be able to translate, what we are experiencing at the other levels of our being. Our intellects are linked to our personalities, which is the surface stuff and relates to how we operate in this world. I personally like striving for cognitive understandings of phenomena as best I can. It is advantageous to have intellectual understandings, especially when we are presented with novel concepts. It helps us to ground our understandings into the context of our reality – as we go about re-creating our reality.

We have to dig deep to reach those aspects of our consciousness that are connected to universal consciousness, to have a more profound understanding, or should I say, *experience,* of existence. This might well require that we get beyond our rational mind for a while, yet not lose our grounding in our agreed-upon, 'real' world. Like the shaman who can move between, yet be fully present in, different levels of reality or 'worlds', without losing his or her grounding in the conventional world.

Our fear of the unknown wants us to cling to the familiar and have a rational explanation for phenomena. The familiar reinforces who we think we are and our place in the world; and that makes us feel safe at a personality level. Even if it also makes us feel miserable. We cannot really fear an unknown we have not yet experienced. We are just re-hashing our known fears and projecting them onto future worst-case scenarios. Maybe the unknown is much, much better than what we have already experienced.

Sometimes we have to concede that there is no rational explanation for certain phenomena and we might surrender our wanting to know to 'mystery'. I would like a dollar for every time I have heard people say to me "You are too much in your head". I also know there are deeper aspects of myself that align more with mystery, and seek more of the mystical; though I do not necessarily reveal this side of myself. I guess that the fear, and the call to surrender, is to be 'out of my mind', to lose the control of trying to make things safe, predictable, known and rational.

Conclusion

In health-care the emphasis is very much put on the tangible, what we can perceive through our five senses; and this of course is supported by the scientific method. The vast interconnecting reality of *consciousness,* which underpins every other phenomenon, is generally considered irrelevant – *if* it is considered at all.

We are so accustomed to perceiving reality in a certain way that to look beyond our agreed-upon version of how life works often takes a radical shift in understandings and perceptions. Most of us are a long way from accepting and exercising the power of our own minds, and our more expansive consciousness, particularly when we are facing health challenges. We easily default to our habituated way of thinking, our customary beliefs, when stressed. We cling to familiar concepts and procedures, even if there is a better way.

When you instil the habit of becoming familiar with your *own* mind you will become aware of how it so influences your personal reality, including your health. This can be extrapolated to the power of thought in general. Rather than thought being a nebulous by-product of the brain, it is the channelling of consciousness, from which everything else springs forth. Your own consciousness, aligned with a benevolent universal consciousness, can be your greatest healing tool.

End of Chapter Points

- *We are currently de-programming some of the old programs that no longer serve us, that have proven to not be life and wellness enhancing.*

- *We are rapidly expanding our understanding of the role **consciousness** plays in every aspect of our lives, including our health and wellbeing.*

- *The 'holistic' model of health recognises that consciousness plays an integral role in health and illness.*

- *We are re-discovering the ancient wisdom that **thought** creates, or at least strongly influences, our experience of reality.*

- *Brain and body are the downward (yet concurrent and not separate) manifestation of **mind**, which is part of the more expansive **consciousness**.*

- *Thought has great transformative and creative power so it is to your advantage to use it wisely.*

- *Particularly, our bodies are constantly responding to our mind-content, most of which is subconscious.*

- *The **subconscious/unconscious mind** has a lot to answer for! It is much vaster than the conscious mind and is well and truly in the driver's seat regarding our health and very lives.*

- *Many people are now recognising that **mind/consciousness** is the 'great untapped healing tool'.*

- *The practise of modern medicine is based on the **Newtonian** model of reality, which views matter, including our bodies, in mechanistic terms.*

- *The **Holographic** view is that everything is interconnected and that a part of a whole reflects the whole. This can be extended to how our mind-body works.*

- *It is when we misinterpret life, and superimpose our judgements upon our human experience, that the body will react in kind.*

- *Strong intention combined with strong emotions can move mountains.*

- *Science has its brilliance and we should avail ourselves of its beneficial developments – but we need to see it in the right perspective.*

- *The intellect might never understand, or be able to translate, what we might be experiencing at other levels of our being. There might always be an element of 'mystery'.*

Chapter 3 | Energy Medicine

"If quantum mechanics hasn't profoundly shocked you, you haven't understood it yet."

NIELS BOHR
(1885-1963, DANISH PHYSICIST)

What is 'Energy'?

We tend to think of 'energy' as this nebulous, intangible substance that does not have the credibility of hard matter. We have decided to give credence to the physical world of matter because it is tangible. We can see it and touch it – therefore it is real. Generally we cannot see or touch energy, though we can perceive its effects. We know that it has many forms such as electrical and magnetic, and that we use it externally and internally continuously. We know that different types of energy have many applications in modern life and the world of science.

The literal meaning, and the general understanding, of the term 'energy' is: force, vigour and activity – the force applied to move matter. We know the aim of our biochemistry is to produce energy to fuel the physiological processes that maintain life. Energy also refers to the by-product of the metabolism of our food: the energy currency of our cells – ATP (adenosine triphosphate).

When we say that someone has a lot of energy, we are stating that they have significant vigour with which to actively participate in life. When people are energy-depleted, they obviously have less capacity to contribute to, take from, and engage in life.

In accordance with classical physics, we know the movement of charged ions across cell membranes create electrical currents (action potentials) that are conducted along nerve cells to enable their functioning; and that the movement of ions contributes to the functioning of so many other physiological processes within the body. Energy is involved in much, if not all, of our body's processes and is an integral part of all living things.

We are aware our hearts beat continuously because of a rhythmical electrical impulse (the pacemaker) that arises from a group of cells called the sinoatrial node, which is embedded in the musculature of the right atrium of the heart. As there is no obvious extrinsic neurological control of this mechanism, we still do not know what starts this electrical impulse we are so reliant on. We know that in the foetus the heart develops before the brain.

Energy is generally described in terms of 'vibration', 'frequency', 'waveform' and 'amplitude'. Vibrations are oscillating motions around a fixed position and they tend to be regular and periodic in nature. Frequency is the speed at which something vibrates, i.e. the number of waves passing a point in a certain time. This is measured in hertz (Hz.).

Waves are formed by a disturbance created by a vibration within a medium, and travel from one point to another within the medium. The amplitude refers to the size of the wave and is a measurement of how much energy the wave is carrying – the greater the amplitude, the greater the energy. Energy is transferred in the direction in which the wave is moving.

Generally speaking, the higher the vibration of an energy form, the more ethereal it is; and the lower and denser the vibration the more it is aligned with matter, including the matter of our bodies. Our human system has many levels of energy, ranging from the lower, denser to the higher (or 'subtle') vibrations, at any one time.

Energy is termed 'gross' or 'subtle'. *Gross* energy abides by the classical laws of physics and is measurable by traditional scientific means and perceived through our five senses. *Subtle* energy is beyond our usual means of detection, such as through our five senses, and is therefore deemed non-existent by many.

Vibration

We live in a vibrational universe, meaning that everything, all phenomena, at its base level, is made up of energy. We are translating energy *vibration* through our senses continually. We are interpreting energy through our senses and translating this into the experience of our reality. In fact, we are so good at it that we are usually totally unaware of the process.

Various energy frequencies are detected via our senses, and thus our nervous systems, and then translated into our perception of our supposed 'outer' reality. For example, when we are listening to music, we are often not cognisant that we are interpreting the energy frequency of harmonics. To most of us music is just *music*. When we see an object we are interpreting photons of light that hit the retina at the back of our eyes. Our physical world is not separate from the world of energy. They are totally interconnected, interdependent and superimposed upon each other. It is all a matter of perception.

We understand that atoms are the basic building blocks of matter and that atoms are made up of protons, neutrons and electrons and various other subatomic particles. Quantum physicists have discovered that when matter is broken down to smaller and smaller particles, those particles no longer have the traits of objects. It has now been well demonstrated that subatomic particles, such as electrons, can behave as particles or as waveforms (energy).

These subatomic particles, or 'quanta', will not be confined to one form, and this has been shown to be dependent upon the observing consciousness. From this it has been deduced that the observing consciousness is not separate from what is being observed.

Here we are entering the world of possibilities and probabilities rather than that of linear cause and effect. Of course quantum theory disturbs our conventional view of how reality works. It is potentially changing our world-view, our core understanding of reality and how we can interact with it.

The theories of entanglement and non-locality add further to the intrigue. They are based on the understanding that there are no completely separate parts and that all in the universe is connected and in a potentially immediate way. It is understood there is no actual distance within this connecting field. Thus, a thought can have an instantaneous effect that is not impeded by physical distances or time.

Advanced theoretical physics has demonstrated that everything in the universe is at some level connected to, and interdependent with, everything else; and that there is a field of energy beyond, yet interwoven with, the world of form. In accordance with this *holographic* view of reality, we can appreciate that the mind-body is a complex energy system, with there being much more than a linear 'cause and effect' connection between mind and body.

There are many comprehensive texts and studies in quantum physics that will give you more understanding of this fascinating area of science that is pushing our understanding of how life works.

In short, these understandings have been brought to our awareness by the lateral thinking and adventurous exploration of some brilliant minds. They have the capacity to totally change our world-view and experience of reality. It is very exciting that our natural human tendency to explore and grow has helped us to see beyond the confines of limiting beliefs and world-views.

A *reductionist* approach to how our bodies work, and to health care in general, will find no limit in dissecting down to smaller and smaller parts, but at the risk of getting further and further away from the whole.

The Energy of Thought

As previously mentioned, ancient mystical traditions and Quantum physics have come to the same conclusions that thought affects matter, and these understandings can be extrapolated to how our bodies work.

Everything, including thought-forms as well as matter, at its basic level, is energy at various vibrational levels; and all of these energy fields can interact and affect each other. Einstein's assertion that matter and energy are dual expressions of the same universal substance allows some understanding that the *energy* of thought can affect the *matter* of our bodies.

Like everything else, thought is energy. The first law of thermodynamics states that energy does not dissipate. It might change form but it has to go somewhere. We are constantly sending off energy vibrations from our thoughts, attitudes, emotions and beliefs, and this will have an effect within and without. The energy of a thought will draw to it that which resonates with it. It pays to hone our awareness of what we emanate from our being.

Thoughts do not just dissipate but continue to exert their effect. As previously mentioned, strong, repeated and agreed-upon thoughts are very potent indeed and are sometimes termed 'thought-forms'. These thought-forms entrain other similar thoughts, and have a powerful influence upon the tone of our thinking and feeling, and how we operate in this world. A bit like the snowball effect, you could say.

So, the more we control our thoughts and thus our vibration, the more we influence our reality. 'Control' is maybe too strong a word as it implies force. Let's replace it with 'manage'. We do not have to be over-vigilant about this, as the calmer we are, the easier and more gentle the process is. It becomes a positive habit to maintain this awareness, and if we do not, life will give us some appropriate feed-back one way or another.

What has this got to do with Health?

In 'energy speak' it is the *vibration* of our thoughts and related emotions that particularly impact the body. Obviously different thoughts and emotions carry energies that vibrate at different frequencies. We can feel this in our bodies. We know when something does or does not feel good, when the energy is *life enhancing* or *life depleting*.

Our prevailing thought-patterns quite specifically affect our physiology. At the base level everything is energy at different levels of vibration, and it is at the level of energy that everything interacts. So thought interacts with our biology at this subtle energy level, as well as through the brain at a more gross physiological level.

A thought will create a feeling, which has a particular energy vibration that affects the vibration of the physical at a subatomic level. This is then translated to atoms, molecules, organelles, cells, tissues, organs and physiological systems until it manifests at a gross biological level. If this process goes on unchecked it can cause a physiological dysfunction that will produce symptoms if the vibration is not in harmony with the system as a whole.

This relates to our body's feed-back mechanism that will indicate to us, via our body's processes and symptoms, the vibration of our thought-patterns and related emotions. Certain thought-patterns will impede the healthy flow of energy in the body, whereas others will enhance it.

The term 'energy block' largely refers to the impedance of the healthy flow of subtle energy due to unresolved emotional experiences and related thought-patterns and misconceptions about life. As already discussed, when emotions are suppressed or repressed, but still very much alive, they particularly affect our bio-energy systems.

Our bodies respond very specifically to what we think, feel and believe. As stated, it is particularly the *vibration* of our thoughts and emotions that so affects our physiology at a subtle energy level. This is the real area to work on to bring about change within ourselves, our health and our lives in general.

'Energy' and Modern Health Care

Modern health care is based on the biochemical model. Scientific endeavour has developed some amazing understandings regarding how our bodies work at the biochemical level and this has contributed enormously to advances in health care. However, we also need to recognise that the mind-body is a complex bio-energy system and that disruptions in the flow of energy affect the functioning of our bodies.

According to the mechanistic/'reductionist' view of reality, on which traditional science is based, we largely assume that 'external' things are separate to ourselves; that there is no connection beyond a physical, mechanical interaction; that what is experienced within has no influence beyond our bodies.

We generally believe our external reality – the world – has nothing to do with our internal selves; that we interplay with it only through our senses. We assume it is a one-way street rather than a two-way street. Therefore, based on this belief, if we want to effect change in the world, external to ourselves, we can only do so by some sort of action, force or physical means. This extends to health care, where it is generally believed that for any healing to occur something external to ourselves must be applied to bring about change within.

Energy medicine recognises that the body is animated by a universal energy, sometimes referred to as 'Qi', 'chi', or 'prana' – the flow and distribution of which affects our health and wellbeing. This universal energy is equivalent to universal *consciousness*, as consciousness is energy. Our chemical reactions and physiological processes are underpinned by, and interdependent with, our energetic systems. They are just different levels of manifestation, understanding and perception.

Traditional Chinese Medicine and various other healing traditions have long recognised there are energy channels that connect the emotional/mind realm to our body's organs and tissues.

What is the point of these flows of subtle energy through and round our biological systems? It makes no sense that energy flows for energy's sake. There must be a higher order at work. It is understood that energy carries information; information that instructs the functioning of the tissues or substrate on which it impacts, imparting information necessary for its functioning.

Genes affect the body primarily through creating and changing proteins that are essential for the body's structure and function. As far as we know, genes do not organise the whole. It makes sense that there is another system at play, a force or 'field' that has an overall organising effect; a field that imparts information to enable the cells to organise into particular forms, with our genes being but the blue-print.

Like any community, if our cells, tissues and physiological and biochemical processes are working together as a whole, this results in greater harmony and health of the system. We have trillions of physiological and chemical processes going on at any one time. It is understandable that there is a coordinating force – or energy field – to integrate these processes, otherwise chaos would reign.

Our immune system is designed to restore order within our human system, to re-integrate what has been made separate and incoherent by trauma or a host of other factors. Our immune system is designed to bring the body back to homeostasis, and needs good communication and cooperation with other body systems to bring this about. It will work well if there is enough of the right 'energy' with which it can function.

It is clear that seemingly separate parts of the body need to communicate effectively with each other for a well-functioning, integrated whole – just as within a community of people. Trauma, whether emotional or physical, has the capacity to fragment the whole. In fact, it is the fragmentation of the whole. If we have shut off a part of ourselves because of trauma, this will not add to the harmony of the whole until it is re-integrated. Open channels of flow and communication will help to bring together those separate parts.

Anything in life works better when there is communication and coherence, particularly if to a higher order; and it seems that energy is the communicating substrate that underlies all other systems.

Energy Systems and the Human Body

The mind-body is made up of many energy channels, energy bodies and energy fields. These include meridians, nadis, chakras, auras and the 'assemblage point'. Many others have also been described. It also appears that physically, mentally, emotionally and spiritually we are connected with, and informed by, various universal etheric energy fields.

Meridians are 14 distinct energy pathways that carry energy into and through the body. Points along the meridians are where acupuncture needles are inserted, as in traditional Chinese Medicine. The meridians connect with every organ and physiological system in the body. If there is a disruption in the flow of energy through a meridian it can affect the functioning of the corresponding organ or physiological system. Disruption to the flow of energy in meridians can be due to a variety of factors, including blocked or disturbed emotions, nutritional, environmental factors, and so on. Blocked and unresolved emotions particularly lodge in our energy systems.

Chakras are often described as spinning vortices of energy that act as energy stations or transducers of the universal energy entering or leaving the body. Different chakras have different colours that relate to different frequencies. They are the interface between the subtle energies and our physical bodies, between the metaphysical and the physical. They represent aspects of *consciousness* and are closely associated with our endocrine glands and nervous system. Each main chakra is situated in the area of a major nerve plexus. We have seven main chakras, all having different functions, and many minor chakras. Chakras are connected to the meridians.

Chakras hold a record of everything we have experienced in our lives, and each chakra is believed to hold a universal spiritual life lesson. It is our task to work through these spiritual life lessons in sequence for the evolution of our consciousness and the overall health of our system. Chakras can be blocked, open or closed, and spinning in different directions, which can reflect a disturbance in the advancement of our consciousness and can give rise to body disorders. It is the task of the energy healer to detect the imbalances and related causes, and help clear and align the chakras. No doubt they also have a self-regulating system.

Chakras, meridians, and other energy bodies generate a large energy field around the body called the auric field. The auric field has a number of layers extending from the physical plane (closest to the body) to the spiritual plane (furthest out from the body). These subtle energy fields surround and penetrate the body and are linked to the energy environment outside the physical body. As with many subtle energy fields we are still discovering exactly what the auric field is.

The 'assemblage point' is a strong and important epicentre of energy, connected to radiating energy lines and has its entry and exit points in the area of the heart chakra. The appropriate position of the assemblage point is related to health. Trauma, whether it is physical, mental, emotional or spiritual, can cause a disturbance of the position of the assemblage point, which can significantly impair psychological and physical health.

(Since writing the first edition of this book I have been informed that our chakra system, as we understand it, is changing in accordance with the evolution of our consciousness - so what we have previously understood about this energy system might not still apply.)

Energy Healing

'Energy medicine' is focussed on the flows and communications of the various energies that underpin our biochemical and physiological processes, and that connect the mind realm to the physical. Energy healing promotes the flow and harmonisation of energy for a positive physical effect and the overall wellbeing of an individual.

The difficulty with explaining energy medicine is that energy is generally not visible or tangible (although it is to those individuals who have highly-tuned perceptive skills). Some forms of energy are generally too subtle to be detected by standard measuring instruments; however, this is now changing as we catch up scientifically with what has previously been delegated to esoteric understandings.

We are gaining more understanding of the 'non-manifest' behind the 'manifest' – or world of form. Gravity is also not visible but its effects are apparent. We accept the concept of the energy of gravity because we accept the scientific explanation for how it works and it has had time to filter into our belief-systems.

Matter, including the physical aspects of the body, has the densest energy and is the last place where a dysfunction will become manifest. In the world of energy medicine it is understood that changes occur in the energy fields before they reach the level of the physical. Many energy therapies are aimed at affecting the *subtle* energy before it is translated into a physical effect.

Energy healers learn to work beyond their personalities and tap into a higher consciousness or broader field to most benefit their clients. They understand that they are transmitting energy from this broader field rather than using their own.

We can also influence our own energy fields, as *thought is energy* and we can learn to become aware of and adjust our own thought-patterns. The energy we put out, related to our thoughts and emotions, very much affects our own body. When we bring our presence (our consciousness) to our own bodies, in a positive way, we promote health. Feeling and becoming acquainted with the energy of your own body and related fields can be a very beneficial meditation practice.

When we instinctively rub a sore or injured spot we are applying healing energy to the area. When you think of your big toe you are sending energy to it in one form or another. It pays to inhabit our bodies with positive aspects of our consciousness. Everything responds well to the right sort of energy.

Our energy extends beyond our skin surface and can interact with that of others as well as with the general environment, near and far. Our field can interact with that of another without any physical touch. It has been well demonstrated that the heart energy extends well beyond the borders of the physical body. In fact, it has been demonstrated that energy can be 'non-local' so our range might be very far indeed. Energy healing at a distance is based on the understanding of 'non-locality' and the immediacy of the field of consciousness.

Ultimately all *healing,* and all therapies to that affect, are to raise the energy vibration – *to raise the level of consciousness.* It is all a means to evolve our consciousness.

Vibrational Therapies

Energy medicine understands that our energies are also impacted by other energies such as electromagnetic fields, other environmental influences, other people, and so on; as well as what we hold in our own minds. Vibrational therapies are designed to affect the various subtle energies within an individual, as well as influence the effect that other energies (environmental, etc.) might have *on* an individual.

Many of these energy therapies cannot be explained, nor verified, in biochemical terms as they are working at a completely different level to that of biochemistry. Energy is *energy*, even though it is interconnected with and will impact the physical, including the chemical levels of our bodies.

Some vibrational therapies have been misunderstood, and often scathingly dismissed by those proponents of the common scientific method. Therapies such as acupuncture evolved over thousands of years and were refined by extensive empirical knowledge and strong intuitive knowing of what worked. Do we better trust what has evolved and been trialled over millennia; or, the results of scientific studies? I would say a combination of both.

Many natural therapies work at a subtle vibration/energy level and this is where they have their therapeutic effect. Herbs, essences, aromatic oils, homeopathic remedies, etc. have specific vibrations that interact with the energies of the human system. The particular vibration of the herb or essence will have a specific impact to balance the energy of the recipient to promote health. Nature worked that out and was not at all interested in 'proof'.

In modern times we have tried to glean a scientific explanation for how these agents work, and that is valid in its own right. A biochemical explanation is not mutually exclusive to an energy-medicine explanation; however, I believe that we are in danger of missing the point if we focus only on chemical aspects. Underlying all biochemistry is energy. They occur concurrently and interdependently. We now know that molecules interact through their energy fields rather than just through physical interactions.

In current times herbs are often used like pharmaceuticals, but they are not pharmaceuticals, they are herbs and work at a subtle energy level. We know that many pharmaceuticals are derived from plants and herbs, and that the *energy* of the plant – how it really works – is often shrouded in a more commonly accepted pharmacological/chemical explanation.

Energy carries information, and in the healing context this information is to promote coherence, and thus health, in the recipient. Various plants, herbs and minerals carry a specific energy signature related to the qualities of the agent. For example, a resilient plant will transfer an energy signature related to the quality of resilience for the benefit of the recipient.

Okay, I admit it, I love crystals. I write this with a little trepidation as in some arenas it is assumed that those who relate to crystals are totally out of touch with the real world and beyond redemption; that they are card-carrying hippies and ageing flower children that live in La-la land. I notice how even those with broadened views who are operating on the edge of mainstream like to publically be derisive of crystals – just to let everyone know that they have not completely gone *off* the edge.

I love crystals not just because they are pretty things but because I have at least a little awareness of the vibrational power and information they hold. Crystals and minerals have individual energy vibrations that can specifically interact with the energy of what they come into contact with – for healing. Crystals are not just girly things. I have seen many very masculine men work beautifully with crystals. The new generations of individuals coming to Earth appear to be much more in touch, in a natural way, with the power of crystals and they will teach us much.

We so easily overlook the healing gifts of nature that might reside in our own backyards and that are gifting us with their energy information.

Kinesiology

My interest in energy medicine was ignited when I studied kinesiology. My studies in kinesiology have given me insight into, and acceptance of, the world of energy, particularly as it relates to our human system. It helps me understand the mind-body connection at its base level. I see no conflict between describing phenomena in terms of, say, biochemistry, and in terms of energy. To me they are different levels of manifestation of the same universal substrate. (I understand that the term 'kinesiology' can refer to different health-care disciplines. In my country – Australia – it is an energy medicine health-care discipline, not a muscle physiology health-care system.)

Kinesiology is the science, and the art, of energy balancing, using muscle monitoring as a biofeedback tool. Kinesiology is based on the principles of Chinese Medicine in combination with many techniques derived from the chiropractic system. It is a non-invasive health-care discipline that deals with aspects of mind, body and spirit as it is based on the understanding these areas are interconnected, and thus influence each other.

Kinesiology does not diagnose or treat medical conditions/diseases but facilitates healing through energy balancing. Kinesiology recognises that there are flows of energy within the body that relate to every tissue and organ, and that connect the mind/emotion aspects to the body's physicality. It is about balancing the energies to optimise the healing process, to 'put the power back on', so to speak.

'Balancing' means relieving blockages to optimal energy flow and addressing the underlying causes of the blockages. These include nutritional, structural, environmental, genetic, emotional and other causes. The energy imbalances can be evaluated by muscle testing, which allows access to the body's overall state of structural, chemical and emotional balance. Muscle testing will guide the practitioner to where the corrections need to be made.

The client will let the kinesiologist know, through muscle testing, what specific imbalances are present and what specific awareness and corrections he or she needs as a priority at that particular time. Through muscle testing, the practitioner is directly communicating with the subconscious mind/body of the client and bringing what is relevant to conscious awareness.

It is particularly kinesiology's biofeedback technique that provides the practitioner with the opportunity to access and communicate with the client's subconscious mind. This is where the programs that run our lives reside. The subconscious mind holds all of our beliefs, attitudes, repressed emotions, and has a record of everything we have ever personally experienced, as well as our ancestral and broader influences.

Bringing to conscious awareness our subconscious programming allows recognition that some of these programs do not serve us well and allows the choice for change. Awareness weakens the grip of negative belief-patterns and allows more empowering new decisions to be made. Learned and inherited programs are often the root cause behind illness and dysfunction, as is unresolved trauma.

In kinesiology we use the term 'life energy', which refers to the amount of energy one has to work with to resolve a problem or issue. If there is low 'life energy' it can be an up-hill task until this is restored to a reasonable level. The whole aim of a kinesiology balance is to restore the client's life energy by detecting and addressing energy drains and blocks, and harmonising the flow of energy through the system.

It is understood that our biochemical and physiological processes, and thus organ function, will work more efficiently when our energy systems are balanced and healthy.

I have met many master kinesiologists and I am in awe of their ability to combine the best of science with the best of the more esoteric disciplines, and deal with aspects of mind, body and spirit at the same time. It truly is a holistic health-care discipline.

Entrainment

Entrainment is when nearby objects synchronise their energy oscillations – e.g. grandfather clocks in a room together. It has been measured that the energy from healer's hands are at particular frequencies that entrain the energy of the client. The intention of the healer, and the receptivity of the client, enhances the process.

Healing in this fashion best draws on a higher energy that is independent of any personalities involved. The information imparted with the energy is to trigger healing in the recipient's system. The process might well involve bringing to awareness, and resolving, the blocks that might lie in the way.

I have often wondered if a person can passively heal another. I believe there must be some resonance and willingness on the part of the recipient in order to be healed, with the recipient drawing the right person/healer to him or herself in accordance with their own intent to be healed. As we are not really separate from others, nor from reality in general, it makes sense that there can be a transfer of energy from one person to another; and particularly if it is drawing on energy beyond the personalities involved.

It might well be the willingness or resistance of the recipient, and even the healer, that might enhance or impede this flow of universal energy that has the capacity to heal. Correct intention is an integral part of energy healing. Intention is a thought, backed by a strong emotion. Thought and emotion are *energy* and will impact the object of intention.

And what *is* healing in this context? It is the transfer of energy from a higher order to entrain that of a lower order, to enhance the coherence and overall health of the recipient. The more coherent and harmonised a system, the healthier it is. It is understandable that a chaotic and fragmented system is less healthy and whole. A person who has a higher, more coherent energy, will potentially entrain those whose energy is more fragmented, just by their presence alone.

However, I do believe that the recipient/client does have to exert some effort to implement the changes. It cannot be a completely passive process. A large part of any energy therapy, including kinesiology, is to bring to the client's attention things that they might need to address and change in themselves and their lives.

In accordance with the understanding that energy underlies everything, entrainment will also be happening at the atomic/molecular, then cellular and organ level. Entrainment to a higher order within a system will promote coherence of energy and unification of function at its many levels – and thus health.

Human Interconnectedness at an Energy Level

We are evolving to recognise and experience our connectedness to the collective, and this will be reflected as our communities become more global. We are linked to others at an energy level as well as at a societal level.

Though we operate as individuals, we are very connected to humanity as a whole, especially our family of origin, our ancestral line and groups with whom we align. Energetically, at least to some extent, our energies are intertwined and we are influencing each other, at conscious as well as subliminal levels, constantly. Two people sitting in the same room (or even miles apart) will have their energies interacting whether they are aware of it or not.

Everything we do, and even think, contributes in some way to the whole. It is sobering – but maybe enlightening – to know that everything we think, feel and do, contributes in one way or another to the collective. Some might refer to this as 'all is one', and this is a concept that makes perfect sense to me.

We are constantly and usually unwittingly bouncing off our issues with each other as well as contributing to the learning of each other. Like rough stones colliding on the shoreline, we will have our rough edges smoothed off by these human interactions life provides for us. We are each, individually, contributing to the *collective* growth and evolution. Sometimes it pays to not take our personal journey – so *personally*.

Like it or not, we are inextricably linked to our family and ancestral line, clearly at a physical level through our genetics, but also at a broader energy level. We tap into the 'field' of our ancestral line. 'Miasm' is a term that was coined by Dr Samuel Hahnemann, founder of homeopathy, and refers to inherited energetic imprints or tendencies that work at a subtle energy level. It is a term generally used in the context of vibrational medicine and homeopathy. These inherited tendencies – *miasms* – will manifest and potentially cause illness in response to certain triggers to which an individual might be exposed.

These miasms are related to unresolved emotional issues and blocks in the evolution of consciousness in the ancestral line, and can create illness, if triggered, in the descendants. What we do with our ancestral, and even broader human influences, is up to us *individually*. We, as individuals, have the opportunity to heal what we have inherited; and some might believe the healing will extend backwards along the ancestral line, as well as forward.

We can even, at an energetic level, take on other people's 'stuff'. There is a kinesiology term called 'surrogation', which refers to a situation where one individual, energetically and unconsciously, takes on another's emotions. This often happens with family members or others to whom one might be emotionally close.

There must be some resonance with the particular emotions they take on. This is, of course, an unconscious process.

Particularly, a child can unwittingly take on the energy of their parents/care-givers' issues out of a mistaken need to relieve them of their suffering. It can also be the child's unconscious attempt to relieve their parent of their emotional burden so that the parent might be more present and available to care for the child. This is a no-win situation for all involved and individuals might not realise their involvement in this dynamic, and how it has so affected them, until many decades later.

In terms of human interactions there is much that goes on below the surface of our conscious awareness. It pays to know what is yours and what is not; and that what is not yours is for the other to work through as part of their life path.

We can be aware of an energy – good or bad – between ourselves and another and be confused as to where this comes from as it is often not related to the interaction at a personality level. The interaction at a personality level might be telling a certain story; however, our 'gut', or intuition, might be giving us very different information. It pays to know ourselves well so that we can better understand what is coming from us – our own 'stuff', and what we are tapping into from others.

The more that we are centred in and know ourselves, the less we might be affected by external factors. The contrary is also true in that the more we are tuned in energetically, the more 'sensitive' we might be to other energies. So we need to find a balance between being centred in ourselves, yet not cut off from, and sensitive enough to, the energies that surround and interact with us.

I believe that at a deep level of our being, and in accordance with 'all is one', what we perceive in others is at some level a reflection or projection of what is within ourself. It is not always necessary or appropriate to work at this level consciously; however, our human systems are working on this regardless. When we work on ourselves we are benefitting the collective; and when we do not, it also affects the whole, particularly if we maintain unconscious habits that might not serve us well.

The Energy of Intuition

"Don't let the noise of other's opinions drown out your own inner voice." ~ Steve Jobs

We all know intuition exists and we all use it, whether we acknowledge it or not. In fact, we use it so much, it often remains at a subliminal level, unrecognised. The *knowing* of our intuition informs us at a level beyond our intellect. You know when someone is staring at you, and you look around to see a person at the other end of the room looking your way. In fact, the knowing is so rapid that it bypasses the intellect and you have already, by reflex, turned around as a reaction to that awareness before the intellect registers it.

That 'gut feeling' is very real. We are not trained to tune in, and are generally very distracted by the busy-ness of life with our focus largely on external things. If we were to tune in we can easily be aware of how our own energy and our body responds to certain people, places and situations. This is not at all to make one paranoid regarding what can get them from the illusory outside, but to encourage one to know themselves well; to be well acquainted with their own inner world so they can learn to harmonise their external environment with their internal needs as best they can.

We have all had experiences of knowing when someone is going to call. Many people have dreams of events that happen at a later date. I have certainly experienced this. I have a large tree in my front yard and I remember dreaming a large branch of that tree falling off and thudding to the ground below. I did not think much further about that brief dream – until the event happened, just as in the dream, and the very next day.

One might argue that I had discerned the branch was due to fall and my dream had brought to light what my subconscious, or 'intuition', knew. Consciously, I had given that tree absolutely no thought at all and there was no suggestion the tree might drop a large branch.

I recall a friend of mine dreaming in technicolour detail, with all the emotional content, of losing his job. The exact event played out the next day – unexpected, apart from what the dream had indicated. How can that be? Was the event pre-empted by, and the circumstances thus attracted by, the tone of the dream? Or, was he tapping into the field of information beyond time? There is no rational explanation within the context of linear time.

It seems our inner knowing, our intuition, taps into a field beyond (though inclusive of) our rational understandings. It is *knowing* without *thinking*. It is our connection to the universal intelligence, what some might refer to as the 'superconscious mind'. That connection is honed through our life experience and all of our learning. We refine our intuition by acting on it – or not – and noting the feedback that we receive. The fundamental quality that underpins the utilisation of our intuition is *trust*.

Medical Intuition

Humans are capable of many levels of perception, some more than others; however, it appears that we have collectively closed down much of our deeper perceptive ability at the altar of agreed-upon intellectual understandings. Clearly there are those individuals who have the capacity to read energy way beyond what most of us are capable of. They can tap into that larger field of information.

Some people are gifted with, or have developed, a very special level of perception that enables them to detect beyond the ordinary. They have different antennae that allow them to pick up energy signals that bypass most of us. For example, some people can pick up the energy traces on objects from a previous owner, or can pick up the energy in an environment related to events previously played out in that environment. We tend to be suspicious of this quality because we do not understand how it works. Frankly, it frightens some people.

I have had the good fortune of meeting many people with these gifts and have absolutely no doubt they can tap into energies, realms and dimensions beyond our usual perceptions. Because their skills are so finely tuned and out of the ordinary, there is often no verifiable 'proof' of the level of subtle energy they can detect. We commonly do not have the tools and capacity to measure these finer levels of energy. That does not mean they do not exist.

There is an area of health care called 'medical intuition', where individuals use their expanded perceptive skills to read the energy of people as it relates of their health concerns. They can often visualise energy and can detect blockages and distortions that relate to certain experiences the client might have endured and that remain unintegrated and thus unresolved. They can tap into a time line to determine when certain events were experienced and how these affected the individual and contributed to their current health issues.

It is said these skills can be taught; but from what I have observed, it appears some people are just born more gifted in this area than others. Experience over time will develop the skill and we probably all have it to some extent.

The area of medical intuition has not yet gained acceptance in the conventional health-care world, as it is hard to fit into the medical model and currently accepted ways of doing things. I have no doubt, however, that practitioners of various health-care disciplines use their intuitive and highly tuned perceptive skills in their day-to-day health-care work. I look forward to the time when these skills gain more general understanding and acceptance.

Beyond Normal Perceptions

For deep healing to occur we sometimes need to enter into the world of 'non-ordinary reality' – the world beyond, but interwoven with the world of our usual perceptions. Much lies under the surface of our conscious minds and it takes specific skills and techniques to access these areas. These skills are usually developed and honed over considerable time and are aimed to heal forgotten and hidden parts of ourselves. These hidden parts can span the ages and dimensions and lie well below the tip of our conscious minds.

Individuals often intuitively know if some aspects of themselves are not yet healed. The language of our conscious minds often cannot access the vast, deeper parts of ourselves. One has to go beyond the intellect to reach these areas that remain hidden and unhealed but which still exert an enormous influence on our wellbeing, our behaviour in this world, and often our health. There are currents within us that go much deeper than our surface attitudes, though our surface attitudes and present dysfunctions might lead us to them.

As mentioned, there are some practitioners who are particularly skilled at seeing beyond our normal perceptions and into other realms of our existence. They are often referred to as 'medical intuitives', 'shamans' and 'healers'. They might have insights into why one might have a particular physical or emotional issue that a Myers-Briggs assessment or biochemical test might not reveal. In short, this area does not fit the medical model.

We are much vaster than we perceive. Long-forgotten and buried experiences can be recalled, in a safe environment, to be resolved, forgiven, integrated and healed. These experiences always have relevance to one's current reality. These processes help us to remember that ultimately all we experience is for our growth and evolvement, and they help us to tap into our natural, but often long-forgotten, peaceful state of being.

Energy and Environment

"The microbe is nothing. The terrain is everything."

It is said that Louis Pasteur (1822-1895) made this statement on his deathbed; and that the quote originated from Claude Bernard (1813-1878), a contemporary of Pasteur. By his alleged statement Pasteur put to question his germ theory that had pointed the cause of disease to microorganisms invading the body and playing havoc with the body's systems.

This statement suggests it is not the microbes themselves but the *environment* the microbes come into contact with that is most important regarding the causation of disease. We tend to think of bacteria, viruses, and other pathogens as invading our hapless bodies, particularly if we are stressed, our immune systems depleted, or we are in the wrong place at the wrong time.

Could it be that these organisms are responding to the vibrational signals our cells are emitting, and that this in turn is related to the energetic vibration of our thoughts and emotions. 'Like attracts like'. When we work on our internal 'terrain' – mind and body – the less we will be subject to these external influences.

When there is an epidemic, possibly the collective community is attuned to certain thoughts, beliefs, attitudes and feelings that are not consistent with health, and those individuals who link into these are therefore vulnerable to the infection.

If one is allergic to a substance, we know that within the body there will be a cascade of chemical and physiological reactions to the allergen and this will produce some uncomfortable symptoms. Might the said allergen – for example a food – have an energetic signature the body perceives as threatening and thus responds by heightening the immune response? Might food eaten when one is experiencing a particularly potent emotional stress be then linked to that stress and perceived as harmful to the body when later ingested?

When we take people, kinesiologically, to when they had the onset of an allergy, we often uncover significant emotional stresses or events that occurred at the time when the offending food was being ingested. The subconscious mind links the food to the particular stress and thus perceives it as a threat, mustering an immune response whenever it later comes into contact with it. "What about genetically inherited allergies?" you might ask. These emotional stresses, if significant enough and unresolved, can influence our genes and thus the allergies that we inherit.

Our energy ('life energy') is responding all the time to our internal and external environment. It has been demonstrated that people universally respond the same way, energetically, to different external stimuli – when viewing paintings or photographs, for example. Some stimuli prove to be life enhancing (they raise our 'life energy'), and others life depleting (they lower our 'life energy'). Though there might be some individual susceptibility, there are overall trends we are all subject to.

Feng shui is the science, or art, of adapting the environment (for example, of a building or dwelling) so that it best harmonises with the individuals who inhabit that environment. The aim is to positively enhance the 'life energy' of the inhabitants, by means of optimising the flow of energy in the environment so that it is conducive to the flow of energy within the individuals. This will create a 'constructive convergence' of energies.

Conversely, 'geopathic stress' is where individuals are adversely affected by the energies of a particular environment or location in which they spend some time. This might be related to a disturbance of energies – subtle and gross – due to such things as underground mineral deposits, underground water courses, various geological energy lines, electromagnetic radiation, and so on. We are interacting continuously with the environments in which we find ourselves.

There are also various other sources of energy we might come into contact with that might not be conducive to our wellbeing. These include energy traces left behind from previous events that have taken place in that environment, and from previous inhabitants. We often know if an environment is conducive to our wellbeing or not. I am sure you have had the experience of walking into a building or room, or onto an area of land, and knowing whether it is in harmony with you or not; compelling you to either linger or make a hasty retreat. Other people are also part of our environment.

As previously mentioned, the more we are centred and healthy in ourselves – physically, mentally and spiritually – the less adversely affected we will be by these other energies that we might come into contact with. The more we know how this works at a rational level, the less fear we will have regarding these phenomena. Interest and curiosity puts us in a much better place than fear. Those with more finely-tuned radars will be much more aware of various other energies, but they do not necessarily have to be adversely affected by them.

The more that we, individually, contribute a positive energy to an environment, the more the whole will benefit. It is to the advantage of all for us to do our individual bit in raising the energy and being aware of the influence of our thinking patterns and intent on our surroundings. Japanese physicist, Dr Masura Emoto's famous experiments on water have well demonstrated the effects of thought, intent and prayer on the energy structure of water molecules.

This can be extrapolated to the effect of thought, emotions and intent on our internal and external environments. As our bodies are mainly water, and our tissues have a crystalline structure, it is understandable that thought and intent can have a direct effect on our biological systems, as well as on the environment we inhabit.

Conclusion

The world of energy has not yet been given the nod in the conventional medical world, even though we utilise it in much of our medical technology and know that it is an integral part of the functioning of our mind-bodies. However, as we evolve our collective human consciousness and our understandings beyond, yet inclusive of, the biochemical model we are gaining more understanding of this fascinating area of health science.

I equate *energy* to *consciousness,* and its various forms and flows with the myriad information that consciousness imparts. Energy underlies and connects everything. This makes more sense from a holographic perspective.

What has previously been relegated to esoteric, mysterious and implausible domains of healing will be accepted as the new medicine – the medicine of the future, as we get clever enough to work out the logic of its intricacies. This involves moving beyond the mechanistic version of how life works and conceding that underlying what we perceive through our five senses is a vast and connected world of energy.

Energy is not bound by time and space, and we can move it with our hands, and with our minds and hearts. As we learn to understand and manage this energy, it will have great impact on health care and our very experience of life.

End of Chapter Points

- *Everything, including thoughts and matter, is energy at different levels of vibration.*

- *Einstein's famous E=MC2 allows some understanding that energy and matter are the dual expressions of the same universal substance.*

- *We need to think of thoughts as 'things', because at an energy level, they are.*

- *The higher the vibration of an energy form, the more ethereal it is; the lower, denser the vibration, the more it is aligned with matter, including the physicality of our bodies.*

- *Matter, including the physical aspects of the body, has the densest energy and is the last place where a dysfunction will show up.*

- *We are interpreting energy through our senses at every moment and translating this into our experience of our reality.*

- *In 'energy speak' it is the vibration of our thoughts and related emotions that particularly impact the body. Our bodies respond very specifically to what we think, feel and believe.*

- *Energy medicine recognises that the body is animated by universal energy, sometimes referred to as 'Qi', 'chi', or 'prana'; the flow and distribution of which affects health and wellbeing.*

- *Ultimately, all healing, and all therapies to that affect, is to raise the vibration – to raise the level of consciousness.*

- *Energy or **vibrational therapies** work with the body at a **subtle** energy level.*

- *With energy healing, **universal energy,** transmitted through the healer, entrains the energy of the recipient to a more cohesive, higher, and therefore healthier form.*

- *The correct intention is an integral part of energy healing.*

- *Our energies are intertwined and we are influencing each other at subliminal levels constantly.*

- *The more we are centred in and know ourselves, and balance our own energies, the less we will be adversely affected by external factors.*

- *We all use intuition, whether we acknowledge it or not. That 'gut feeling' is very real – trust it!*

Chapter 4 | Beliefs

"If you don't change your beliefs, your life will be like this forever. Is that good news?"

W. SOMERSET MAUGHAM
(1874-1965, BRITISH NOVELIST)

Our beliefs are the perceptual lens through which we view the world. We generally believe the world is static and that everything 'out there' is perceived in the same way by everyone. It is not. We all live in our own little worlds. We all perceive life through our own filters, based on our beliefs.

Our beliefs run us, and influence our experience of life. In fact they create our experience of life. Our thoughts and beliefs do create our reality. What we believe is true – for us, but not necessarily for others who do not hold to the same beliefs. Our beliefs will draw to us, in terms of life experience, what is consistent and resonating with them.

Everything we do is determined by the priority of our beliefs – *everything*. Beliefs are the bottom line! Thus we do not have 'free will' if we are run by these subconscious beliefs – our 'programming'. We kid ourselves that we do, but we don't as long as this programming is controlling us from behind the scenes. Becoming *conscious*, meaning aligning with aspects of consciousness beyond our conditioned ego mind, will allow choice.

Like a fish that does not notice the water it is immersed in, it is similar with our beliefs – unnoticed in our background consciousness. We take them so for granted they usually sink into our subconscious mind, controlling us from their hidden position. We usually do not question or even examine our beliefs until a life situation might force us to do so. It is particularly our life experience, as well as appropriate education, that will adjust our beliefs over time.

Our beliefs are related to thought-patterns that are so habitual they get 'hard wired' into our neurological system. Like wheels that slide into ruts in the road, our thoughts easily go down those neurological pathways structured by our beliefs. It is a continually reinforcing process. We are continually and unwittingly *proving* our beliefs, which will, of course, reinforce them. Beliefs are like self-fulfilling prophecies. It is an ongoing process until we gain some awareness of it. This is both an individual and collective process.

Beliefs have a strong emotional component. They are very visceral and are how we emotionally condition the body. As previously mentioned, suppressed/repressed emotions hold our beliefs in place and once we release the emotions the beliefs are less rigidly held. Tuning into our emotions and feelings will give us an inkling as to what underlying beliefs are being triggered.

Underlying any ongoing 'negative' emotions are certain thought-patterns, perceptions and, particularly, beliefs. These are the basis of why we react as we do. Dealing with the core, and often misconstrued beliefs will help soothe the emotional reaction. It also goes the other way around in that releasing our suppressed emotions will uncover and help adjust the related beliefs.

The problem is that many of our beliefs do not work well for us but are maintained out of habit and because we do not consider an alternative. When we experience our suppressed emotions it opens the opportunity to bring our underlying beliefs and related thought-patterns to the fore. Our emotions will lead us to the beliefs we are harbouring in our subconscious mind. When we are aware of our subconscious-mind content we can apply our will and determination to alter aspects of it. That is the name of the game.

When our beliefs are put on the table we can decide whether they serve us and whether it is beneficial or not to maintain them. We cannot do this if we do not know they are there. We have the opportunity to change our beliefs and attitudes if we are *conscious* of them. When they are lurking in our subconscious mind, assumed and unexamined, we will not change them. Of course we also have many beneficial beliefs – it is best to keep those.

When our beliefs and related thought-patterns are not aligned with the natural flow of life and our natural selves this will cause us pain and dysfunction at some level; and this is designed to give us appropriate feedback to help us question those beliefs and put us back on track. Our bodies will give us feedback regarding our beliefs, one way or another. We sometimes call this illness.

Life experience, awareness and education weaken the grip of negative belief-patterns and allow more empowering, life-enhancing beliefs to be adopted. By the process of feeling our emotional reactions to our life experiences, resolving any related trauma, and examining the related negative beliefs, we start the process of disempowering them. Of course this takes some willingness, training and discipline. It takes some persistence to instil new habits of thought, and thus change those disturbing beliefs.

Where do our Beliefs come from?

Our beliefs come from myriad sources including our 'programming' from our 'tribe' (family, society, school, workplace, etc.), beliefs held by the collective consciousness in which we are immersed, and our response to (how we interpret) our individual life experiences.

The collective consciousness, what society has *agreed* upon, has an enormous influence on what we individually believe. Our family, group and society's beliefs are extremely compelling. Humans are very impressionable and therefore easily programmable. We often listen to the loudest or most powerful voice – the great 'They'.

We want to be included and accepted by our communities and our survival does depend on this to some degree. We do not want to look different by having ideas and notions that rock conventionality. We are often very suspicious of new beliefs because most people are threatened by change and what is outside the 'status quo'. It can be very inconvenient!

We know that throughout the ages some very courageous individuals challenged the status quo of prevailing belief-systems. Many scientific beliefs, held as sacrosanct at one time, later proved to be incorrect and were upgraded; for example, genetic determinism. If we did not push beyond what we already knew, we would not be driving cars or have put aeroplanes in the air.

It is particularly our early-life experiences that have such a major effect on what beliefs we formulate and maintain. It is not the experiences per se but how we *interpret* those experiences that instil certain beliefs. It is our way of trying to make sense of the world by putting our experiences into some sort of rational context (though beliefs are often *irrational*). It is also our way of trying to keep ourselves safe by establishing some sort of consistency and 'ground rules' for life. Beliefs are our hard-wired thought-patterns about how life works.

Various healing modalities, including Kinesiology, might 'age recess' a client to take them to a time when a belief was formulated or adopted. I recall during a session a woman remembering when, as a young child and in response to an experience, she believed she would never have children of her own. She recalled the exact moment of affirming that belief which, although consciously forgotten, was still having a significant influence on her those many years later.

At a deep, subconscious level we base our survival on our adopted beliefs, and thus we will often not relinquish them readily. Our beliefs are our reality and our understanding of how we survive it; thus they can be exceedingly tenacious.

Suppressed, repressed, unexpressed emotions, thoughts and feelings are related to past experiences that remain unresolved and unintegrated. In response to certain experiences, particularly when experienced at a young age, we develop certain beliefs and attitudes about ourselves, others, and life in general. We might then develop various defence mechanisms and learn to conform in ways that remove us from our true selves in an attempt to gain acceptance from the 'tribe' and protect ourselves from perceived harm.

It is the non-acceptance and non-integration of certain life experiences, and the resultant defence mechanisms, that create an emotional charge that keeps these beliefs in place. In addition to causing some dysfunction in our lives in general, this process can potentially affect our physiology and cellular function and culminate in organ dysfunction and illness.

There is very often a significant emotional release when the hammer is hit on the nail of a dysfunctional belief. Out with the old, in with the new. Release and integration of the related emotions will help move the energy blocks that hold the beliefs in place. Objectifying our beliefs after the disturbance in emotions is healed, loosens our attachment to them and thus their power over us.

Beliefs and Behaviour

Beliefs are like the central nucleus from which emotions and behaviours spring forth. If, at a deep level, you believe you are inadequate or unworthy, you will sabotage your much-wanted success for fear it will put you in a position of proving your inadequacy or unworthiness. Self-defeating behaviour will be an ongoing pattern.

Unravelling this process starts with acknowledgment and acceptance of your humanness in having this pattern, and then intending to adjust your beliefs to align with a healthier outcome for yourself. It also involves allowing yourself to feel and integrate those related emotions that you might have tried hard to avoid.

One could say that beliefs are conditioned states of mind from which we are trying to predict an outcome. The way we see the world is actually based on our prediction of how we see the world, based on the beliefs formulated from our past. When we predict our future based on beliefs that have been developed or acquired from our past, this leaves little room for change, novelty and growth. Our assessment of the now, and our expectation of the future, is based on beliefs derived from what we have already experienced.

When I was a child I had an experience of being bitten by a dog. This occurred when I was walking to a friend's place (as we often did unaccompanied in those days). As I was setting out I remember feeling excited as I was anticipating an outing with my friend. As I was happily walking down the road, a dog suddenly ran out of a yard and bit me on the leg. The bite was very painful and left me feeling shocked, afraid, vulnerable and angry.

When we react with shock we quickly suppress any emotions and then unwittingly formulate beliefs to make sense of the experience and as an attempt to ward off further similar experiences. It is our way of trying to keep ourselves safe. One of the beliefs I formulated, for a short time, was 'all dogs are dangerous'. I was avoidant of all dogs for some time but eventually dispelled that belief when life provided me with the lesson that not all dogs are dangerous.

However, it was many years later when I realised that the belief I had developed from that experience was *'if I am anticipating something happy I will be blocked by something painful'*. It was not about dogs at all but a belief that had a much deeper and more profound effect on my life and potential to sabotage my happiness. That belief was related much more to my *feeling* sense of the experience than to the physical circumstances, and it might well have reactivated a similar prior belief.

I had made a quick but profound (and incorrect!) conclusion about that experience and had tucked it into my subconscious mind, from where I generalised it onto life. That belief remained in my subconscious mind, away from my conscious awareness, but from which it ran the show. My mind had decided that belief was going to keep me safe – from disappointment – but it had the opposite effect.

When I shared that experience later in a workshop, a young woman who was an attendee approached me. My story had triggered a long-forgotten memory in her, related to herself having been bitten by a dog when she was a child. She mentioned that for most of her life she had difficulty looking people in the eye. When she did she had an irrational fear of being attacked by them. As she was setting up a business, this was inhibiting her success.

As I related my story she remembered when, as a young child, she had looked a large dog in the eye just before it bit her. She quickly saw the connection and was able to disempower that belief that had been holding her back from much of what she wanted to do in her life.

Conditioned Beliefs

A belief can be like a 'curse'. Giving someone a set prognosis of a medical condition can indeed be like 'pointing the bone'. Even believing that 'it is in the genes and I therefore cannot do anything about it' can be a self-fulfilling prophecy. Particularly regarding health, we are subject to collective beliefs that have a huge influence on the unfolding of our health challenges. Diagnoses and prognoses come with their inbuilt beliefs regarding expected outcomes. Upgrading our beliefs allows some flexibility regarding illness outcome and the potential to heal.

Particularly the word 'cancer' conjures up all sorts of fears and projections to worse-case scenarios. The word can trigger marked emotional reactions related to what we collectively believe about it. When one hears the word 'cancer', as related to themselves or their loved ones, their whole world changes within seconds, even though nothing else in themselves or their lives has changed within that time frame. The word has that much clout.

The word 'cancer' holds much power in the context of modern health care. The collective belief in cancer very much influences how patients and health-care practitioners deal with this area of health care. The tendency is to take the 'fight it' approach, which is fuelled by the emotional reactions governed by our collective beliefs.

We would not be changing beliefs that serve ourselves, and humanity, well. We would only question beliefs that cause pain and suffering. Of course there are many positive, life-enhancing beliefs and it pays to hold onto those. We are influencing each other all of the time and we can be inspired by positive beliefs, one of which is: *It is possible.*

Often in the sporting arena, when an athlete achieves what had previously been considered impossible, others will quickly follow suit as it has been demonstrated that it can be done – the belief has been upgraded. We might believe that something is not possible until it is demonstrated by others that it is. This can also be extrapolated to how we can be inspired by how others deal with their health challenges. It pays to seek out the stories of people who have defied agreed-upon beliefs regarding illness outcome.

Can we Change our Beliefs?

We do have the power to change our beliefs if they are not working for us – unless we want to hold onto the belief that we cannot. I am not pretending it is easy or even desirable to change them quickly as we feel at a deep level that our survival depends upon them. However, it is at least about being aware of what can so control us.

We have the power to scrutinise and determine whether maintaining certain beliefs is in our own and the collective humanity's best interests. We have to first become aware of what beliefs we might be holding. At least in part, our personal experiences and the life process itself will be up-grading our beliefs. Our life experience includes the influence and education from others.

To change our beliefs we have to change what we know, often including our very selves; and the ego self can have a mighty resistance to doing this. It might take time and persistence to retrain our brains and minds to new beliefs. Changing beliefs can feel like letting go of the handrails, like having the very foundations of our life slip from under our feet. Therefore patience with ourselves, and others, is paramount. It can be very unnerving (no pun intended!) to change our beliefs – yet ultimately very liberating.

It can indeed be very humbling to change what we have held so dear. As the Zen parable about the overflowing tea-cup suggests, we need to be open to releasing our tightly-held beliefs before allowing new concepts and understandings. And these too will change in time, as does all phenomena. Sometimes we just evolve beyond certain beliefs. They just do not fit us anymore and our emotions and intuition (or our body if we ignore these) will indicate this.

It can be a lonely journey if society at large is still holding onto the beliefs that we, ourselves, have outgrown. It is a time to really tune-in to our intuition and the knowing of our inner selves. Even though millions might still agree on something that we can no longer align with – *to thine own self be true.*

Conclusion

It can feel very disempowering to realise that our programmed and adopted beliefs might be working in opposition to our *conscious* intent. When we really have a strong intent to do, be, or have something, and if this is aligned with our highest good, then the power of our intent will, one way or another, overcome those beliefs that might be working against our conscious desires.

So don't give up! Know that our subconscious mind, where we hold our beliefs, can come around with determination, and that 'Life' will conspire to bring this about.

The bottom-line belief is: 'Is life on your side and all that you experience for your growth and evolvement to a better way?' or: 'Is life unsafe and you have to be on guard, and use force, manipulation or compromise, to survive it?' Beliefs are but thought-patterns and these thought-patterns determine our experience of life.

Can we use our minds to determine a reality beyond the conditioned beliefs that can keep us herded like sheep? No longer is it adequate to think life just happens *to* us. We are evolving the understanding that our thoughts and beliefs project out to affect our reality, our very experience of life – and certainly our health.

End of Chapter Points

- *Our beliefs are the perceptual lens through which we view the world.*

- *Our beliefs create our experience of life.*

- *We are continually and unwittingly **proving** our beliefs.*

- *Underlying any ongoing 'negative' emotions are certain thought patterns, perceptions and, particularly – beliefs.*

- *Our beliefs will directly affect the working of our bodies and our health in general.*

- *We have the opportunity to change our beliefs and attitudes if we are **conscious of** what they are.*

- *Many of our beliefs do not serve us well but are maintained out of habit and because we do not consider an alternative.*

- *Awareness weakens the grip of negative belief-patterns and allows more empowering, life-enhancing beliefs to be adopted.*

- *Though our beliefs come from many sources, it is particularly our early-life experiences that have a major influence on what beliefs we formulate and maintain.*

- *It is the non-acceptance and non-integration of certain life experiences, and the resultant defence mechanisms, that create an emotional charge that keeps these beliefs in place.*

- *Putting our beliefs on the table and objectifying them, loosens our attachment to them, and their power over us.*

- *A belief can be like a 'curse'. Giving someone a set prognosis of a medical condition can indeed be like 'pointing the bone'.*

- *Of course there are many positive, life-enhancing beliefs and it pays to hold onto those.*

- *Our bottom-line belief is: 'Is life on my side and all that I experience is for my growth and evolvement?' or: 'Is life unsafe and I have to be on guard to survive it?'*

Chapter 5 | Stress

"It's not stress that kills us, it is our reaction to it."

Hans Seyle
(1907-1982, Austrian-Canadian endocrinologist)

'Stress' is a term that has been coined in relatively recent times and is familiar to most people. Stress refers to the demands on a system, in our case, on our psychological and biological systems. Stress occurs when the demands upon a system are more than the system can cope with. 'Stress load' is cumulative physical, environmental, emotional and psychological stress.

Generally speaking, the greater the demands are, the greater the stress. The body's stress *response* will generally react in the same way regardless of the source of stress. We get stressed when we get too much of what we don't want or too little of what we do want.

Stress and fear are inextricably linked. All stress taps into our fear of not surviving, physically or psychically. The human primal fears that underlie all stress are: fear of annihilation, fear of rejection and abandonment, and fear of the unknown. These fears are all variations of the one theme and boil down to a deep ego fear of not surviving. Bottom line.

Stress and the Autonomic Nervous System (ANS)

Hans Seyles' famous three phases of stress are: 1) the 'acute' phase of stress; 2) the 'adaptation' phase; 3) the 'exhaustion' phase. There are specific physiological and emotional effects related to these different phases.

Physiologically, the *acute* phase of stress puts us in 'fight or flight' to help us do what we need to do quickly to survive what triggered the stress. At this stage our focus is very much on fighting, fleeing, or freezing, in an attempt to survive the threat at hand.

In the *adaptation* phase, we adapt to the sustained stress that we now do not feel we can control or change. We 'bunker down' for the long cold winter and our physiology changes accordingly. We believe the stress is unrelenting and we cope as best we can.

In the *exhaustion* phase, we feel we can no longer cope with the stress and 'throw in the towel', so to speak. The body then goes into degeneration and breakdown as the mind goes into depression. The mind-body has given up the fight.

Physiologically, stress is a catabolic, energy-depleting state. It is highly adaptive in the short term but can have devastating effects in the long term. We all have our predispositions as to how we, mentally and physiologically, cope with stress.

The 'autonomic nervous system' (ANS) is the part of the nervous system that regulates the functioning of our organs and physiological processes that are not under conscious control. For example, the beating of our heart and the functioning of our gastrointestinal tract are managed by the autonomic nervous system, without any conscious or voluntary control. We do not have to think about these processes as they work automatically.

Other body systems, such as our endocrine/hormonal system, play a large role in the functioning of the body's physiological processes, and work hand-in-hand with the autonomic nervous system.

There are two main branches of the autonomic nervous system – the 'sympathetic nervous system' (SNS) and the 'parasympathetic nervous system' (PNS). The SNS gears the body up for emergencies by utilising the 'fight or flight' system; and the PNS calms the body down for rest, repair and recovery.

People can be either SNS or PNS dominant; meaning their default pattern when under stress might be either to speed things up and use energy (SNS) or slow things down and conserve energy (PNS). You can see that some people, when under stress, get active and busy and others will slow down and withdraw.

There are many variations of this and it is not always clearly one or the other pattern. Of course these tendencies have their genetic and environmental influences, and they are not necessarily set in concrete. Ideally the SNS and the PNS are in balance, with activity and energy utilisation being balanced with rest, repair and recovery. When we are more aware of our constitutional types and tendencies, we can better manage them.

What Drives our Stress?

Many of us operate with ever-present feelings of pressure, anxiety or even burnout, and consider this normal. The pressures of life – jobs, relationships, financial pressures, raising children, global events – have become such constant companions that many of us operate with ever-present tension. Stress can be unflagging and we often accept this as a standard part of life.

Many of us feel guilty if we are not racing around and being constantly overactive. There can be a constant feeling that there is never enough, that we must strive for more and maintain the competitive edge; or that *we* are not enough, and have to achieve more to prove that we are.

Stress indeed can be addictive. We become reliant on those bursts of adrenaline to energise us to do what we feel we need to do. We might even become suspicious if we are not experiencing that adrenaline drive, as subconsciously we have associated our very survival with it. We might experience a perverse sort of comfort when experiencing those adrenaline surges as we equate them with our ability to survive the situations at hand and life in general.

The mind is a major culprit when it comes to stress. Yes there are environmental stresses, and so on, but we usually cope with those one way or another. Mental stress, as governed by our beliefs and patterns of thought, can be unrelenting and constantly putting us in a state of stress. We can be either regretting or re-living the past, or projecting onto a fearful future. As we tend to focus on the mind, we can easily over-*think* rather than *act* when it is required. Movement will dissipate those stress hormones, as in the animal realm; but over-thinking will keep us in a stress loop.

Why are we so driven? Why is there relentless busy-ness for most people? If you have ever driven on a freeway you know what I mean! The pace of our lives seems to be exponentially increasing, as is the information load. Our society's value system is based on what we achieve and the image we put out. We believe we need to 'look, be, do and have' to a certain level to be accepted by the 'tribe' – our community – and thus keep our place on the planet. These modern-day survival fears drive much of what we do.

Our early life impressions and programming influence how we feel we need to 'look, be, do and have' to ensure our place in the tribe. This will make us very prone to stress if we feel we are not living up to those standards and demands as dictated by others and society as a whole. This is usually an unconscious process that is very influenced by the messages taken on in those early, formative years.

Stress is caused not so much by 'not coping' but by thinking that we *have* to. "If I do not cope, what will *they* think? How will I be judged by self and others if I cannot do what I said I would?" This again goes to our deep rejection/survival fears. This can even lead to depression, underlying which can be significant self-worth issues that have been triggered by these circumstances. The mind-body might then withdraw from active engagement in life, in its attempt to survive, and this can manifest as certain illnesses, particularly the fatigue syndromes.

Look at what attracts the rewards in our society. Is it wisdom, kindness or integrity? I think not! What is glossy and on show and driven by competition and aggression clearly gets more kudos, at least superficially.

There is nothing wrong with any of that, or with being driven to a certain extent. It becomes a problem when you base your self-worth, and by extension your survival, on these achievements. When you are driven by how you think other people want you to be – or not be – you will create stress by removing yourself from your intuitive directives of what is best for you.

Having a sense of purpose and meaning in life, and clarifying one's values, will put one in a more stable position from which they will be less influenced by the opinions of others and society as a whole, and less thrown by the vicissitudes of life.

People can be very busy and have many demands on them but not necessarily feel stressed if what they are doing is in alignment with their real needs and wants. There might be some temporary stress but this is not a cause of suffering as it is experienced in the context of an overall purpose. It is when we are motivated by trying to survive, which essentially means trying to prove our worth to others and society, that we will be more vulnerable to stress.

We will also be more prone to stress if we have only assigned things in the external world as a means to our happiness, fulfilment and worth. When we re-discover our inherent power to determine our own experience of reality, we will be much less subject to stress. If we believe that our health can only be influenced by external factors, rather than our inner dimensions, we will feel more vulnerable.

A significant cause of stress is feeling trapped and disempowered. When we feel disempowered we tend to believe we are victims to an external world in which we have to fight hard or manipulate to survive, or completely resign to. Whereas, if you believe all that you experience is ultimately for your benefit (and I do know this is a stretch sometimes!) and that life is on your side, you will be more relaxed about the unfolding of life. Particularly when you believe you, yourself, are the main factor regarding your experience and the out-working of your life, you will be less prone to stress.

Stress and Subconscious Programs

One of my greatest stresses in the past was when I had 'car trouble'. This was particularly when I had young children, was stretched and stressed anyway, and did not feel supported by life. The dreaded 'car trouble', in my mind, meant I could not continue with my daily routine, could not get to work, had to drain finances, which meant I could not put food on the table and pay the rent, and therefore my children and I would be on the streets and basically not survive.

Of course this did not happen; however, my mind, in the flash of a second, went through that scenario as if it did. It was all mind-generated and way out of proportion to the reality. Similarly, being caught in traffic and late for work can have us reacting like we are running from a tiger. It does not seem like a great deal on the surface but can be enough to tap into our subconscious primal survival fears, pending our past experiences, mind-set and circumstances at the time.

When stressed and *unconscious* we can easily default to our habituated patterns of thinking and behaviour. The emotional/limbic part of the brain has the propensity to react with alarm to what it perceives as a threat, at the expense of the brain's higher, more rational functioning. The frontal lobes are bypassed and the brain loses integration when it reacts in this alarm fashion. It takes some training to use the higher aspects of the brain to overcome this default mechanism that so easily puts us in 'survival mode'.

I am often intrigued that even when I intellectually know I am safe, I can observe my body (thus my subconscious mind) go into the stress reaction in response to certain triggers. That part of me that reacts is running on old programs and does not have the understanding my intellect does. It is working at an entirely different level. Knowledge and insight can certainly help; however, the intellect can do just so much to reach that hidden part as it can be like oranges trying to communicate with apples.

The intellect can acknowledge and attempt to understand those parts of ourselves that are running on old programs and trying to keep us safe. It is tempting to reject that part, but I think that approach never helps, as it impedes integration by further shutting down the part that is trying to have a voice. It might take some considerable mind training to overcome these programs, while at the same time soothing and integrating those aspects of ourselves that have been controlled by them. Meantime it is a matter of learning to live with them and manage them as best we can.

The stresses we are subject to are not always obvious. They can be subliminal, away from our conscious awareness but very much held in the body. We can unwittingly hold the stress of unresolved experiences from our past in our subconscious mind, and thus our body, for years. These can fly well under the radar of our conscious awareness but have profound effects on our emotional and physical health.

These subconscious stresses are potentially more of a problem, particularly regarding the effects on the body. When stress is apparent to us we can deal with it; but when it is subconscious we are unaware of what can be causing us harm. There will, however, always be some manifestation from the mind-body holding stress, and this is often in the form of physical symptoms. There are a number of healing tools, including kinesiology, which can help one access the subconscious mind where these subliminal stresses lie. Meditation can be very helpful in accessing our subconscious mind content.

Stress can result from subconscious beliefs such as believing we are not worthy of receiving the good that life has to offer; and that, therefore, we will miss out on having our needs and wants fulfilled. These fears drive us to attempt to gain what we might subconsciously believe is not our due; so we are fighting against the resistance that is fuelled by those beliefs. This scenario can be associated with regret and guilt for not having achieved what we believed we should have; and this belief causes our sense of self-worth and self-esteem to plummet further.

Our stress can be related to believing we cannot fulfil our potential and do what we are here on Earth to do. Well the truth is that we are doing it anyway – life will always, one way or another, be pushing us in the direction we need to go; and feeling stress might well be part of that push. Our stress might be related to our not experiencing what we would have liked to experience in life, forgetting that *all* of what we have experienced is for our growth. We need to be reminded of the perfection of our lives.

These beliefs, that cause us so much stress, are countered by the understanding that we were always going to make the decisions about our life that we did, given what we knew and our level of development at the time. We are not missing out on anything, as *life* will deliver to us exactly what we need for our growth and the development of our wisdom. Our consciousness will get what our consciousness needs, and this is not always in accordance with what our ego wants. And as for our worthiness, we need to be reminded that is a given, our *birthright* – no matter what.

This does not mean you sit back and do not get on with your life. Of course you make plans, follow your desires and make appropriate adjustments to your life. You do what you want and need to do. However, if life does not go according to your plans, if anything unexpected comes your way, it helps to see that there is a purpose and learning in this. Life is such that it is always, one way or another, leading us in the right direction, with this process being streamlined when we align with that universal intelligence rather than the dictates of our ego minds.

Stress and Loss of Brain Integration

When we are stressed we might lose *brain integration*, meaning that the different regions of the brain do not communicate with each other as they might do when in a non-stressed state. Put plainly, when you are significantly stressed, your brain, temporarily, does not work as well as it might at other times. People can feel confused, scattered and split-off. You might recognise that fuzzy-brain feeling, sometimes called 'brain fog', when under stress. You just know that everything is not working as it should. This is because the more primitive 'fight or flight' mechanisms of the hindbrain take over at the expense of our frontal lobe, executive brain functioning.

Children are particularly prone to loss of brain integration when under stress and this can lead to learning and behavioural problems. It is said that successful people are particularly skilled at maintaining their brain integration when under stress; therefore they function well when others might not. The aim is to reman centred despite any external chaos and this is a skill that can be learned. There are some simple stress-relieving techniques that can be very helpful to maintain or restore brain integration, particularly if employed early enough.

Stress and Regression

If one has unresolved early-life stress, this will stay in their system and be reactivated by certain life situations that, subconsciously, remind one of the original stress. When this is the case, one can regress, emotionally and in the moment, to that earlier age when the original stress was experienced. This can be associated with a mild shock-like state and it can be very difficult to respond appropriately to the situation when in this state. This is when we react rather than respond.

I have certainly experienced this myself and have sometimes caught myself going into this state, or later, in retrospect, have realised that this had occurred. I have learnt to catch myself when I feel myself regress – awareness does help. When you feel yourself going into that 'brain fog', regression or shock, try to pause and remove yourself from the situation as best you can. Calm yourself and then let your rational, adult mind regain sovereignty. This is not a good time to make decisions. And please note, some people are very skilled at observing this state in others and using it to their advantage.

It really is a matter of the adult you learning to calm that scared inner child that is freaking out (yes, like it or not, we all have one and it pays to introduce yourself to him or her). Awareness is the key; and this involves getting to know yourself at a deeper level and understanding your own individual stress-reaction and triggers. The inner child needs to know that the adult is in charge. Sometimes we might over-compensate and bring forth that warrior energy to protect that inner child.

I had known Melissa for many years. I met her initially when she was utterly overwhelmed after having had her first child. She had a very child-like demeanour and appearance and, despite being a very conscientious mother, was having great difficulty in looking after her new baby girl. The slightest thing out of her routine would set off marked anxiety. She was particularly anxious about her baby's health and welfare. Melissa was diagnosed as having post-natal depression and spent some time, with her baby, in a local mother-baby unit. This initially helped and put her into a more comfortable routine.

Melissa had had a very strained relationship with her own parents, particularly with her mother. It appeared that some of her emotional development was halted by her early-life experience and her family-of-origin dynamics; and the stress of having a baby triggered those unhealed parts. She clearly regressed to a child-like state when under stress; and her over-conscientiousness and anxiety reflected this.

When one is markedly over-conscientious and over-responsible this is often due to their being run by that overwhelmed inner child, whose emotional development, in response to certain experiences, was halted at that early age. That child aspect often lives in fear of being *punished* if not acting according to what is sanctioned by society at large. This can cause one to adhere to rigid routines and often anxiety is triggered when that routine is interrupted for whatever reason.

Melissa's condition gradually improved with various therapies, though she was still prone to bouts of anxiety when under stress. Ongoing counselling with a very skilled psychologist, appropriate treatment, and adopting good self-care greatly helped her. As I saw her over the years I could see her adult self gradually gain dominion over that frightened inner child. She gradually became much more empowered with a greater sense of self.

I observed Melissa change from someone who was almost incapacitated by anxiety to someone who appeared to genuinely enjoy life and have healthy self-trust. She was much better equipped by the time she had her second child; and she also proved to be a great help to others by sharing what she had learnt through her own experiences.

Panic Attacks

We definitely have our individual predispositions to stress, and this very much relates to what we have experienced in the past, and how we have reacted to those experiences. If one experienced significant stress in their early years, the stress response can become like a hair-trigger that is easily set off. Your intellect might be well aware that there are no significant current threats yet the body might react as though there is a life-and-death struggle going on. This is because the subconscious mind, which works hand-in-hand with the body, and which is associated with the more primitive, 'survival' aspects of the brain, over-rides the frontal lobe functioning at these times.

'Panic attacks' (as opposed to ordinary anxiety attacks) characteristically occur when people are feeling relaxed and cannot identify any immediate threats in their current environment. This is because something that might appear banal, and not even be consciously noticed at all, has triggered a significant unresolved stress in their subconscious mind. What might appear to be completely harmless to the conscious mind has been perceived as a major threat by the subconscious mind. Phobias work in a similar way – they are *representative fears* (such as fear of spiders) where the conscious mind has not recognised the *real* source, which is a significant unresolved fear from the past.

Therapies that try to relieve panic attacks or phobias by getting the client to face their fears by employing graded exposure (e.g. to spiders) do absolutely nothing to deal with the underlying issue. They might help the surface fear, but at the risk of driving the underlying unresolved fear further underground.

Degrees of Stress

We can confuse a small amount of stress with excitement. They feel very similar in the body and it depends upon the interpretation we put on these feelings. Those butterflies in the stomach can arise when you are anticipating something new and exciting or when you are dreading the unknown and projecting worst-case scenarios. Better excitement than fear. Why don't you get excited about the unknown and new adventures, rather than dreading change? If one door closes, maybe a better one will open. Some change in life is inevitable so you may as well embrace it. The fact is that you would not grow and evolve if there was not some change.

Our society often confuses stress with weakness, or 'not coping', and thus we tend to suppress, deny or distract ourselves from the feelings of stress. That is all fine to a degree; however, addictions can become our means of distracting ourselves from what we do not want to feel. It is strength that allows us to show the soft and more vulnerable sides of ourselves and this allows others the same freedom.

Soldier on! Deny any human vulnerability! It is actually courageous to admit you have too much on your plate and cannot reasonably do it all – particularly if it is not aligned with your real needs and wants. Not in any sort of precious, self-righteous way, but rather in a realistic way. It is much more beneficial to admit your stress, and then find healthy ways to alleviate it, than deny and further suppress it. Sometimes we have to accept our humanness.

If stress is extreme, and one cannot continue with their normal functioning, we might label this a 'nervous break-down'. There might be many other factors involved, including psychopathology such as anxiety disorders, in some people. It takes a trained professional to sort this out. Regardless, these situations can be powerful turning points for people, depending on how they are handled. Sometimes the old patterns have to break down before new, ultimately more conducive patterns, are instilled.

It goes without saying that any prolonged or marked stress should be addressed, preferably with the help of appropriate professionals. It can be very difficult to get any clarity as to how to help yourself and sort out your life if you are feeling overwhelmed. This can be a time to surrender for a while and seek help from those you trust and who are trained to deal with these situations.

Stress is not all Bad

We are all going to feel stress at times. Some stress is a normal part of life and actually of great benefit physically and mentally – to a degree. As is said, 'your greatest growth is when you are out of our comfort zone', when there is an edge of stress. Stress has a valuable function in your life, depending on how you view it. A person giving a speech will be reliant on a little anxiety, as they know it will give them the impetus, focus and energy to perform well. We would vegetate if we did not experience some stress.

It is actually pro-survival to have some stress and over the millennia the experience of stress has helped us adapt to our environments, and evolve and propagate as a species. As is said, 'necessity is the mother of invention', meaning the stress of not having some of our needs and wants fulfilled will drive us to create means to bring this about.

There are physiological benefits to having some, but not too much stress. For example, we will strengthen a muscle by stressing it a little, demanding of it a little more than it was previously comfortable to deliver. Having less food to eat might increase the efficiency of our mitochondria (the energy producing organelles in our cells) to better produce energy from available resources.

We will be out of our comfort zone when we undertake some of life's challenges and venture into new areas of life and change aspects of ourselves that do not serve us well. It is helpful to be reminded that we, as humans, are wonderfully adaptable and resilient. Attitude is paramount, and it is our attitude to all we experience, including the experience of some stress, that is likely more important than the stress itself.

If stress is marked and unrelenting, however, the system might then go into dysfunction and breakdown. If stress is marked it is a warning that something needs to be addressed – either our circumstances, our attitude to them, or both. It is not a matter of just trying to get rid of the stress but understanding *why* we are reacting to our circumstances the way that we are. If stress is marked, professional help is often needed.

Don't Shoot the Messenger

We have tended to collectively make 'stress' wrong. Stress is our indication that something needs to be addressed and adjusted. It would be far more concerning if we did not have these feedback mechanisms, as the underlying damage would be ongoing without the indicators designed to get our attention. If we had a sharp stone in our shoe, we would want to get those pain signals so as to remove the stone and avoid ongoing damage to our foot. As is said – 'Don't shoot the messenger', but listen to what the message is trying to tell us'.

Our bodies know how to do the stress reaction very well and are just doing their job when reacting in this way. This is a good thing if we heed the signals. As with all painful emotions, feeling stress is actually a safety mechanism as it indicates something in ourselves or our life needs to be acknowledged, addressed and adjusted. This might be an attitude rather than external circumstances. It might be dispelling the myths and the programming we have bought into.

The meaning you put on the experience of stress has more clout than the stress reaction itself. It is a bit like the 'fear of the fear' becoming worse than the original fear. Far better to have a stress response than no response if you still have misconceptions about life to iron out. Of course, how you perceive your life experiences, as determined by your beliefs, influences your tendency to react with stress. It is how we perceive the situation, rather than the situation per se, that causes the stress. 'One man's poison is another man's banquet.'

If we reject or misinterpret the signals of stress this is far more likely to cause harm to our biological systems than the body's stress *reaction*. The stress reaction is just the body doing what it is designed to do. It is the causes and perceptions that underlie the stress reaction, and what we do with those, that are more pertinent. The stress reaction is just providing us with feedback on these.

It is never the answer to suggest a person just stops stressing. That can cause more harm than good. There are many pharmaceuticals, natural therapies and methodologies that can help soothe stress. These have their place in calming the system and allowing more clarity with which to proceed with dealing with the underlying causes. However, if the underlying causes are not dealt with, these therapies and methodologies might suppress the stress signals and drive the underlying causes and misconceptions further underground. Potentially, this might then cause illness.

'Better to Wear Shoes than to Cover the World in Leather.'

This adage means that it is better to adjust your own attitudes, beliefs and perceptions rather than try to control all external factors. It really is an inside job. Good luck with trying to control external factors if you see them as separate from yourself. Some would say, and I agree, that we attract life circumstances that align with our own mind content. Some would suggest, and I agree, that there is no completely objective external reality and that all we perceive is largely an out-projection of what we hold in our own mind/consciousness. But I digress into metaphysics.

When you change how you perceive a situation you will reduce the stress. We call this 'reframing'. I know a young man who recently had his driver's license suspended for a time. Usually a very good driver, he was fined for speeding. This occurred on his first day of driving his new car. He might have been a little giddy with the excitement of the newness of it all, having previously driven a 'bomb' for some time. In addition to the suspension, he was also fined a significant amount of money and received demerit points to boot. He had just started a new job and as a result of the suspension there was difficulty with him being able to get to work.

He was initially devastated and had difficulty coming to terms with the situation, as the 'punishment' seemed particularly harsh. Once he settled down and looked for the gifts in this situation, i.e. *reframed* it, he gained acceptance of it and his stress abated. He realised he might be averting a potential car accident by not driving for a while; he would make efforts to be a safer driver after this incident; he was human and could make mistakes; and he had to learn to call on others for help during this time. Also, as he was just starting his career as a young lawyer, this experience might help him to have more empathy for future clients who 'make mistakes'.

An old Buddhist saying is: 'If you have a problem and can do something about it – why worry? If you have a problem and *cannot* do anything about it – why worry?' When you learn to accept and go with the flow of what life presents to you, you will experience less stress in response to your circumstances. This does not mean that you be passive or resigned, or that you do not attempt to change what you need to change. It is a balance between surrendering, viewing your experiences as opportunities for learning, and being proactive about making the changes you might need to make.

At some level, all stress is related to some form of resistance: resistance to the full experiencing of the now circumstances; resistance to uncertainty and an unknown future; resistance to the flow of life; even resistance to life in general and happiness and joy. Resistance means not fully engaging what is. We know how tense our bodies feel when in the state of resistance. Sometimes we need to sit in the eye of the storm and await its dissipation and then clarity.

With acceptance of a situation, comes a diminishing of the stress. With surrender comes relief. As said, this is different to resigning yourself or being apathetic. It is best to allow the feeling of the initial stress emotion, preferably with some awareness, and then allow the acceptance and relief. Like the grief process, one might have to wade through emotions such as fear, sadness and anger before acceptance sets in.

Better to allow and experience those emotions rather than suppress them and cover them up with the facade of 'everything is okay'. Paradoxically, we will disempower our emotions when we lessen our resistance to them, when we mindfully give them our presence. They will more readily be integrated. When we allow (but not *indulge*) those emotions they will more likely move through and out of our system to make room for acceptance to settle in.

If you understand that life will evolve your wisdom by all that you experience, you will be less driven by these survival stresses. Life is on your side, guiding and teaching you all of the time, and when you have trust in this, you will see all of your experiences as opportunities from which to learn and grow. When we upgrade our understandings of how life works, which particularly includes the understanding of our inherent self-worth, regardless of what we do or do not achieve, or how we cope, we soothe the stress reaction.

At the end of the day, wisdom is your greatest ally and it will trump anything else. When everything else falls away, wisdom will be the one redeeming factor you will draw on.

Stress and Physical Health

Now what about the effects of stress on the body, on your physical health? You know that mind and body work together and that ongoing or severe stress has adverse effects on physical and psychological health. That is obvious. However, it is more the specifics of the underlying thought-patterns and beliefs that make one prone to stress in the first place, that so affect our bodies.

The body is taking our mental messages, most of which are subconscious, literally, and is trying to compensate in some fashion. It can be this compensation that gives rise to symptoms, which we might label as illness. The process of experiencing stress will help lead us to the underlying mind content that can contribute to body malfunction.

I do not believe that *stress per* se causes serious illness. I do not believe there is a linear cause-and-effect relationship between stress and cancer. Stress will indeed cause 'wear and tear' and emotional unrest; however, it is just the body trying to do its job. How we handle stress, our conclusions about it, and particularly what in our mind-body make-up causes the stress in the first place, is much more pertinent regarding our physical and psychological health.

Never fall into the trap of trying to remove all stress from your life (impossible anyway!). This process often leads to covering over the related beliefs and emotions, which continue to have deleterious effects on the body. It is much better to look at the *why* behind any prolonged or repeated stress patterns than to go further into suppression. Suppression will just maintain, at a subliminal level, the beliefs and thought-patterns that underlie the stress; and it is these that directly affect our physiology. This, I believe, is much more harmful to the body in the long term. There is a difference between suppressing and *soothing* stress.

Stress and Mindfulness

We can develop the habit of tuning in to ourselves – a form of 'mindfulness', you might say. When you are used to being centred in yourself, you will be more aware of any inner discomfort as it occurs, and get more practised at dealing with issues as they arise. With emotions, when you heed the information they are trying to impart to you, it will prevent them from escalating and becoming distorted. This will prevent you from acting them out unconsciously. Meditation, and reflective quiet time for yourself, are very useful in helping you to get to know yourself.

You have probably all experienced that 'gut feeling' or slight inner discomfort where you know that something is a little off. Sometimes the signals are a lot more obvious, but often they are subtle. Well, I suggest you respect those feelings, as they can be a lot more knowing than your busy intellect. That is 'tuning in' to the wisdom of your own being. Tuning in is innate; we have just been trained otherwise. We have probably all, at times, ignored those inner stirrings only to later find out that it would have been wise to listen to them. This can apply to what foods to eat and what treatments you might resonate with, as much as anything else.

When I am more centred and less distracted by the busy-ness of my life, I will sit myself down if I am feeling that discord and search for the cause. Usually something will become apparent and then I can deal with it. I defuse the stress as best I can. It is when I do not take note of that inner feeling and let my life-demands dictate, that the stress will escalate and often manifest as a physical symptom or emotional upset.

We all know some stress is part of the human experience. Most people will react with stress to certain difficult situations. We can allow some stress, knowing that our mind-body is quite adaptable and resilient. Our stress reaction is very helpful in situations that *do* threaten out survival. It is at times a very appropriate short-term, emergency reaction designed to keep us on the planet. We want it to work well.

It is the underlying thought-patterns that will have a much more deleterious effect on your physiology than the stress response. Suppressing the stress can be one of the worse things that you can do for your body. Alleviating the stress – yes; but not *suppressing* it as those related beliefs and thought-patterns will continue unaddressed. The emotions related to the stress response are our indicators.

Conclusion

The experience of 'stress' brings our attention to what is not working for us. The function of stress is to bring our focus to what is not working in our life, or our own being, so that we can then address and change it as best we can. Our understanding of the stress reaction helps us to *soothe* the stress reaction so that we can more calmly proceed with bringing about the changes that we want. We are in a better position to determine and help *create* a brighter future when the agitation has subsided.

The change might involve altering your perception of, and attitudes to, what you experience. It is not always possible or advisable to immediately change or leave a situation, yet you might develop a deeper understanding of yourself, and life in general, through your experience of it. Looking at the situation differently includes acknowledging what you are gaining and learning from it. When you change how you perceive a situation/experience, you also change how your body responds to it.

It also pays to *intend* a better situation for yourself while you are doing this. The paradox is that when you accept what is, you release the resistance and invite a better outcome for yourself. Acceptance of a situation does not preclude changing it for the better. Inherent in the acceptance of a situation is acknowledgement of the need to sometimes change it.

Sometimes the sensible thing to do *is* to leave the situation. Quit that job or leave that relationship if all other avenues have been explored and you know it is not in your best interests to stay. Only you can judge when the time is best for you to do this and definitely tuning into and calmly following your intuitive leads is helpful here.

Ways to Reduce Stress and Enjoy Life More

- *Adopt healthy habits such as good, nutritious food.*

- *Exercise is clearly stress-reducing unless extreme.*

- *Adequate sleep and rest to allow the parasympathetic nervous system to bring about repair and regeneration of the body.*

- *Nature. We take the simple things for granted. Regular doses of fresh air and outdoor activity. Ideally daily, even if for only 10 minutes.*

- *Find a favourite safe spot and take yourself there in your mind if not physically.*

- *Regular breaks and unstructured time. These can be of short duration if you are busy. They do help to stop the stress loop of our usual busy-ness.*

- *Find an activity, hobby that you are passionate about and allow some regular time for this. Where the mind goes the body follows. Those endorphins and chemicals of enjoyment are very stress relieving and health-enhancing.*

- *Laughter – the best medicine. We tend to take ourselves so seriously. Tension is not great for the mind or body. Let's face it, our human condition can be pretty funny and it is relaxing to make light of it.*

- *Ongoing education, learning and stimulation. Some people get stressed because they are bored and not getting enough stimulation. The world offers so much with which to engage. Learning keeps the mind agile and life interesting. There is strictly no age limit.*

- *Change and novel experiences. We change our habitual thought-patterns by doing new things and experiencing new environments. It helps to get out of the four walls and habitual routine of where we experience our stress. This is not the same as running away.*

- *Spiritual and philosophical interests. Experiencing human life is a spiritual path. We have an innate need to find meaning in our lives. It helps to see our lives symbolically at times and to have spiritual/philosophical understandings to fall back on – particularly in times of stress.*

- *Meditation – of course! It is free and we can do it anywhere, anytime. The benefits are well documented and manifold.*

- *Tuning into your own intuition, rather than other people's opinions, regarding what is best for you.*

- *Treat yourself with love and respect and expect that from others.*

- *KNOW YOURSELF, BE YOURSELF, TRUST YOURSELF.*

Chapter 6

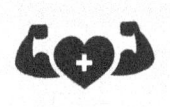

From Victimhood to Empowerment in Health Care

'There is nothing either good or bad but thinking makes it so."

WILLIAM SHAKESPEARE
(1564-1616, ENGLISH PLAYWRIGHT)

The belief in powerlessness and victimhood permeates the whole structure of health care. One of the greatest travesties of truth, that we humans have been programmed to, is that we are powerless and therefore not responsible for our own lives, including our own health. We largely believe we are subject to the random whims of fate or the dictates of a higher power; that we are separate from, but subject to, external controlling forces. If we believe we are powerless then, by extension, we believe we are not responsible for much of what we experience, or more so how we react to our experiences, and are thus subject to victimhood.

Our medical system, our legal system and society as a whole, enables victimhood. There is reward for being a victim and it is often with what some see as the ultimate reward – money. How did we so tie up compensation with money? I am sure the reward of education, for example, would not be so appealing. We have put a value on suffering! Even some people who have lost loved ones, through a means where blame can be afforded, are compensated with money. As if money can somehow compensate for their loss! Someone has to pay!

Victim Mentality

I have personally been steeped in victim mentality. I have had to do a lot of inner work to turn this around; and it is, indeed, still a work in progress. I know very well the seduction of feeling like the innocent, disempowered victim, and of the dependency that goes along with it. This state is quite addictive because, at a subconscious level, it is who we think we are and how we believe we can best operate in the world. In maybe a perverse way, this has made me less empathetic to those who also strongly express this pattern, possibly because I know they reflect what I am aware is in me – and I do not always like to be reminded.

I am very familiar with the ins and outs of the victim mentality and how it can so easily come through the back door when we think we are out of its grasp. I understand how compelling the victim/blame stance can be and the resistance we might have to taking personal responsibility. We all have the victim archetype working in the background of our consciousness at some level, and we will all feel victimised at times.

Some might say the opposite of victimhood is empowerment, which includes standing up for yourself and protecting yourself with appropriate boundaries when necessary. That is certainly the case; but, more so, it is about being *responsible* for yourself and what you derive from all that you experience. It is a matter of seeing your experience of reality as related to your individual perceptions. This understanding does not preclude the necessity of appropriately looking after yourself; you can be aware of the bigger picture while doing what you need to do to look after yourself in your day-to-day life.

One thing I have learnt for sure is that 'Life' does not do pity. At times when I have felt distressed and victimised by certain circumstances in my life I have often called for some insight and understanding – a higher understanding of the situation. The answers will always come, but never as I expect when I am in that frame of mind; they will always be related to an attitude, perception, or something I have to adjust within myself. *Always*. It is never about the other person being wrong or life being unfair, as my ego might have hoped. Very humbling!

If we maintain the victim stance we will see *all* of life through the lens of the victim. There will always be a reason for the victim to be victimised. There will always be somebody or something to blame, someone to point the finger at. When hearing of some tragedy in the news I often wonder how long it will take for the blame to be cast, the class action to be started; and sure enough I will later hear or read of these responses. It has become a conditioned response in our society that there has to be someone to blame for unwanted circumstances and some big brother to come to the rescue.

Victimhood implies: 'it should not have happened; it was wrong that it happened and someone or something did it to me and somebody has to pay; and I had no part to play in the causation.' Victimhood implies that life can get it wrong; that there is a basic design fault. That 'life can get it wrong' is a thought that alarms me more than anything else. I prefer to think that *everything* we experience is ultimately for our growth and the evolvement of our, and the collective's, wisdom; that all adverse experiences are a springboard to a better way. This is not at all denying that bad things happen and should be avoided and dealt with as best we can.

The 'Privilege' of Victimhood

It is much more attractive for some to hold the dubious 'privilege' of being the victim, than to engage the prospect of taking full responsibility and accountability for themselves. It is easier to not look deep within themselves to find the contributions to what they are experiencing. To really recover from an illness, or any adversity for that matter, one has to let go of the victim stance. The idea of personal responsibility is daunting for some. But what would you prefer to hear? That life is unfair, not on your side and that you are subject to the random whims of fate? Or, that you have some personal control over what you experience and particularly how you *react* to your experiences?

Feeling 'victimised' at times is a far cry from taking the victim/blame stance and maintaining it as a way of being and a way of functioning in the world. The victim finds their power in blame and self-righteousness. It is far better to be accountable for your own life and gain the utmost in wisdom from all that you experience. If trauma has been experienced, it is up to us individually whether we choose to heal from the trauma and how we choose to proceed with the rest of our lives. 'Life' does not owe anyone anything. It is what we make of it that counts.

Bree presented to me with a considerably long list of troubling life experiences and circumstances. Her list included ongoing issues with her health and having been "damaged" by a number of surgeries that she had had over the years. She claimed she had never recovered her health following the surgeries and any further medical attempts to help her led to further complications and problems. There was no doubt that she had endured some very difficult experiences and was justified in some of her complaints.

Most of the initial long consultation was taken up with her litany of grievances, and there was a long list of health-care practitioners who had been deemed incompetent or negligent, or both. By the end of that consultation I had a sneaking suspicion I would be added to that list.

She was very offended, and I was accused of lacking compassion when I broached the subject of personal responsibility (after all, probably no-one was *forcing* her to have those medical interventions). Interestingly, when it came to my suggesting health-promoting behaviours such as healthy diet and exercise, there was always a reason why this could not be done. She also frequently presented with a number of different symptoms for which she demanded investigation. I was well aware further medical tests would likely eventually find something that would lead to some sort of medical intervention – from which there might be further complications and reason for complaint.

I find it interesting that many of those who are so blameful and aggrieved by what others have done to them are sometimes themselves the least considerate of their own impact on others. I have seen a number of people who wear their resentment and resultant self-righteousness on their sleeve. They project the message that 'life has done them wrong' and therefore life owes them and should be compensating them for what they have suffered. I have found many of these people to be very self-focused, having the least empathy and consideration for those around them.

It is quite a challenge to help some people when they are filtering everything through the lens of resentment and the belief that other people, and life in general, are not on their side. Their subconscious agenda might be (and often is!) to prove that belief. There is usually an atmosphere of drama and often we have lost before we have started. This situation from a therapeutic point of view can be hard work, yet so rewarding when a breakthrough is made.

Sometimes the doctor is caught between a rock and a hard place when trying to fulfil their duty of care and working within the confines of the medical system. It is a balance between doing what is necessary to follow-up symptoms and address physical concerns while also being aware of the possible undercurrent of emotional/psychological factors. It can sometimes be the classic case of 'the boy who cried wolf'.

I suspected Bree had some significant early, unresolved wounding (which was found to be the case but which she glossed over as insignificant) that was being played out through her dealings with the medical profession. As an authority group we can be subject to patient's projections related to their unresolved issues with their early care-givers.

Sometimes a patient's unconscious agenda is to prove they cannot be helped, that they will again be abandoned and let down. They are unwittingly proving their concurring beliefs, which likely were instilled in response to their early-life experiences. This is a psychological issue that takes great skill from appropriate practitioners to help resolve. Compassion and understanding *are* very necessary components in the therapeutic setting, as is clear communication and appropriate boundaries. Often people just want to be heard and have their experiences validated.

At some level, attitude plays a part in the patient's willingness to heal. When one focuses for so long on what is wrong and not working in their lives they tend of attract more of the same. It becomes such a habit of mind that it becomes very difficult to allow room for what is good and beneficial. Some people are just not ready or willing to let go of their wounds. It can be difficult to tell a patient their unresolved life experiences and related fears, defences and attitudes, rather than tests results and figures on paper, might be the cause of their problem.

We sometimes take a great risk in daring to tell the truth, and I have had past patients who have held vendettas against me for years because of this. My task is then to not myself be victimised by their response. We need to see our attitudes, thought-patterns and beliefs, as the illness in need of correction. We need to depersonalise the process and deal with it without guilt or shame or blame. The paradox is that we also need to see our basic innocence in all of what we experience and what we carry forth from it.

On the other hand, some people develop increased empathy for others through their experience of difficult circumstances, and can indeed become the classic 'wounded healer'.

Alison had also experienced a series of unfortunate circumstances, including significant health challenges and the loss of loved ones. Despite the physical and emotional pain she had endured, she was often cheerful and clearly not focussed only on her concerns. She was mindful and considerate of others. She had made the decision to enjoy life while in no way invalidating her experiences. She took a 'philosophical' approach and shared her gained wisdom. She was willing to feel her emotions fully and receive support, but never presented with an attitude of blame or self-pity.

Teresa suffered from marked anxiety, yet despite this she bravely engaged her life and had a great sense of humour to boot. Because of her anxiety she did experience some significant challenges but would always add a humorous twist when recounting her concerns. I did not feel that she was suppressing her woes; she just saw the funny side of life. She would often have me in gales of laughter, despite my attempts to maintain a more serious tone to the consultation. She often said that she felt better after seeing me; and it was *I* who always felt better after she consulted with me. Rather than going into victimhood and blame, some people just elevate the energy regardless of their personal concerns.

Heather had experienced severe abuse as a child. She was about the most compassionate and caring person I had ever met. She had the heightened sensitivity and intuition that can develop in individuals who live through those sorts of experiences. She cared for others at the expense of herself and this was a pattern she found very difficult to change, even though she knew maintaining it was not in her best interests. Heather had been unwell for most of her adult life. She had a number of debilitating and complicated medical conditions requiring ongoing management.

Some people never allow themselves to feel their grief and anger related to their life experiences, and internalise their distress. Far from resentment and self-righteousness, they might develop marked compassion and consideration for others. At the extreme, however, some people believe they have *no* rights and find it difficult to have healthy boundaries and stand up for themselves in an appropriate way. Their form of victimisation might be that they consider themselves less significant than others and thus put their needs behind everyone else's, believing they are not worthy of receiving due consideration and care from others.

There is a healthy balance between the extremes of narcissistic self-importance and feeling oneself less worthy than others. Clearly the experiences and messages one received in their formative years, as well as their resultant ways of coping and defence-mechanisms, play a large role in this dynamic. Awareness of our entrenched patterns allows us to examine whether they serve us or not. We often need someone else to point them out to us as we will not see them if they have become our habituated way of operating in the world.

It can be a very delicate balance between being accountable for what we experience – what we attract into our arena, and how we react to it, and standing up for ourselves in a healthy way. Being responsible for yourself includes caring for yourself well and ensuring good treatment from others. The evolution of the victim archetype is to cease playing the victim and learning to stand up for yourself in an empowered, healthy way. It includes being accountable for your own life experiences, or at least your reaction to them, and acknowledging the role you have played in them.

At the end of the day, we have to be responsible for ourselves as no-one else can be. This does not mean we do not receive, and give, care and assistance; but no-one can entirely do our lives for us. This includes good health care – we have to do our part. One can have the best health advice in the world but that will be of no use if that advice is not implemented. I recently had a patient arrive for the first time in my consulting room. He had a number of health issues, smoked, drank alcohol to excess, did not exercise and did not eat a healthy diet. He was not prepared to change much of that but demanded that I make him 'better' by July. This was late May!

All Responsibility – No Blame

Many of us have been so conditioned to believe in our powerlessness that those who do hold power can very easily subjugate us. Accordingly, we will transfer blame to those individuals or groups we feel hold power over us rather than hone our own sense of responsibility. People learn to resent those who they feel have power over them. 'Power' is an internal job, and has nothing to do with domination or force over, or from, others.

The victim/blame mentality is sanctioned by a society that loves a victim and dislikes a 'perpetrator', and that does not abide by the philosophy of personal responsibility. This approach encourages the projection of responsibility and personal power to another. Blame can also be a way of avoiding feeling deep, painful emotions, and projecting out what one does not want to really own up to and feel within.

We have been trained to believe that the source of our happiness, and our upset, is external to ourselves. This is fallacious thinking many of us have bought into. When we realise the source of our happiness is related to our beliefs and attitudes, and how we view life in general, we will feel more empowered within ourselves and less adversely affected by the externals.

The belief of the 'law of attraction' (meaning 'like attracts like', and that what we hold in consciousness will attract like experiences to us) is exceedingly politically incorrect and unpopular when tragedy strikes. It is much easier to assume the position of the innocent victim who has absolutely nothing to do with the circumstances they experience in their life.

Does it make sense that an individual has absolutely no influence on, and is in no way accountable for what they *personally* experience in their life, yet another party, who does not even know them, can so easily be put to blame? The word blame should be deleted from our vocabulary. It serves absolutely no life-enhancing purpose. It is based on a misconception about how life actually works.

A few years ago, in my part of the world, there were some devastating bush fires with a large loss of life and property. The amount of loss and suffering was unimaginable and people are still putting their lives together some years down the track. It was in the media recently that class actions were being taken against the local electricity company, the CFA (Country Fire Authority) and various other organisations. People have been straining hard for years to afford blame.

I recall a particular public figure being cast as the scape-goat in this situation. The ugliness of the mob mentality is often added to this sort of scenario. Someone or some organisation has to be made responsible and blamed for this tragedy! 'Someone did something wrong to cause this'. This thinking is based on the misconception of linear *cause and effect*. There are myriad reasons, most of which we are probably unaware, as to why something happens at a certain time. Of course mistakes can happen and we need to learn from them and be accountable for them; however, this is very different to the blame/punishment/revenge *mentality*.

The medical profession, and maybe the health-care industry in general, have been seen as an authority group. After all they have power over your health and your very lives, don't they? Or so you might have believed. When you give a group that much power, you are also likely to give them too much responsibility, and direct blame to them if things don't go according to how you would like. We have paid homage to a belief-system that is the opposite of how life really works.

I cannot tell you how many people have walked into my consulting room and put their health issues on the table and pushed them towards me as though I now have ownership of them. This was often with an attitude of 'what are you going to do with them, because I don't want them any more'. No, they are *your* health issues, not mine. I will do my very best to work with you to help you with your health issues, but their ownership remains with you. I am actually not responsible for them – *you* are. I am responsible for my own, and for giving another the very best health advice of which I am capable.

No-one has ownership of anyone else's health. I consider that individuals are ultimately responsible for their own minds and bodies. I am only responsible for myself, and for my children when they are young; and I have the responsibility to give health advice and facilitate the care of another – as best I can. However, I am not responsible for who another is and what they experience.

People often confuse 'responsibility' with 'blame'. Related to blame is shame, which just increases that sense of powerlessness all the more. It is important to note that when talking about 'mind-body' medicine, the connection between mind/consciousness and health, that it is not a blame game. It is not about blaming one for their physical conditions. *Blame* and *victimhood* are the flip sides of the same coin; and both, in energy terms, are very low on the consciousness scale. Both go together.

It is no help if one goes from blaming outside sources to blaming themselves. It is the same energy coming through the back door and associated with guilt and shame, both of which are disease-inducing. However, it is about gaining insight and understanding, self-awareness and personal responsibility as best one can.

If you do not resolve and integrate your grief, sadness and anger related to an experience, victimhood and suffering can be the outcome. When we don't allow ourselves to feel those emotions as they arise, they will more likely be projected as blame, resentment and even revenge. This dynamic is prevalent in all conflicts, and even contributes to war. Blame, whether of oneself or others, calls for punishment and revenge. And we all know how well punishment has worked in our society!

I am sure that a lot of illness comes about because of internalised blame, shame and guilt. Some would even suggest that personal subconscious guilt underlies *all* serious illnesses.

Of course, any emotions that arise in response to what we experience are related to the underlying beliefs we hold about life.

They are related to the *meaning* we put on our experiences. We are victimised more so by our beliefs and misunderstandings about life than any external circumstances.

The Human Imperative to Care

Many will argue that a small child or an elderly person with dementia or a person with certain disabilities cannot be wholly responsible for themselves. Of course they cannot at a conventional, day-to-day level. It is important to not confuse responsibility with the need for care. Of course care is given where care is needed and it is very much the human imperative to do so.

Here we are talking more about an overview, a larger picture. Every being, no matter what age or state they might be in, is, at a deep level of their being, responsible for the outworking of their own life. This includes (and maybe particularly) the conclusions they draw from their experiences. I have had kinesiology sessions myself where it has been revealed that, in response to certain experiences, I had made profound decisions about my life at age two and a half! These were still affecting me many decades later.

One might say every individual has chosen, at some level, their own life, and ultimately for the maximum growth and evolvement of themselves and the collective. This is a metaphysical, philosophical overview that you may or may not agree with, but one that I hold to and that underlies much of what I have to say in this book.

When people are experiencing difficulties, including health challenges, they should be met with the utmost care, compassion and understanding. Clearly there are those who are more vulnerable and less able to take responsibility for themselves. Their healing might involve surrendering to their circumstances and receiving appropriate care from others. Maybe surrendering and handing over the reins for a time is what is required for their individual healing.

There is, however, a fine line between compassion and pity. There is a difference between caring for someone and attempting to rescue them. There can be a very delicate balance between being fully present with another's distress and vulnerabilities, with compassion, and knowing when to encourage them to let go of their hurts and find the gifts.

Taking responsibility for yourself does not mean you do not ask for help when needed, nor avoid righting a wrong and standing up for yourself when appropriate. Nor does it mean you put up with unsavoury circumstances when they need to be changed. It does not mean you do not experience emotions such as anger, sadness and grief and feel victimised, rejected and betrayed at times. We will all feel victimised at times, and of course we should feel the greatest of compassion for ourselves, as well as others, when experiencing distress.

And of course it is sometimes appropriate to correct an injustice. This can be one's journey to empowerment, as long as one takes some responsibility for the role that they, themselves, have played in the unfolding of their experiences – wanted and unwanted. Ultimately, though, we all have to work on our own point of attraction to all we experience, and particularly what we derive from our experiences.

Cooperation versus Co-dependency in Health Care

A co-dependency can exist between health-care provider and patient. It can suit both parties to maintain an ongoing arrangement where the mutual roles are continually reinforced. 'I need you to reinforce my role as a health-care provider and you need me to reinforce your role as a patient'. This can be a stagnant arrangement with no movement and can promote illness maintenance rather than healing.

It is far healthier when it is a *cooperative* arrangement. The job of the health-care practitioner is to help the client to get to a state where they are not *dependent* on the health-care practitioner, but will seek their advice and expertise when needed. We are all going to be patients at times and the aim should be for this to be a temporary state rather than an identity. (Granted some people do have chronic health concerns that require an ongoing arrangement with their health-care provider.)

The modern health-care system runs the risk of unwittingly promoting the disempowerment/victim stance, which encourages one to look externally, and be dependent on others, for the cure. This is on top of looking *externally* for the cause of the dysfunction. This puts enormous and unrealistic pressure on health-care practitioners and the system as a whole. Obviously external agents and procedures can help to alleviate conditions; however, this should be within the context of primarily promoting *internal* change.

The victim wants both a rescuer and someone to blame. When people are led to believe they are the innocent *victims* of their health issues they often look for a rescuer – the medical profession. They might also look for a perpetrator, someone to blame – often also the medical profession.

Ideally health care encourages the individual to take responsibility for the quality of their health and their lives in general. The responsibility of one's health should be handed back to the client. It is the practitioner's responsibility to provide the very best in information and healing techniques/skills they have available. However, the responsibility for implementing the changes and doing the necessary work is up to the client. This might sound obvious; however, it still is not in the collective to believe this.

How many people go on blind faith and so quickly hand their power and responsibility over to those deemed to have far superior knowledge regarding what is best for them. It seems easier in the short term. When discussing health-care choices I have had countless people who, with almost a child-like innocence, hand the choices right back to me.

I have also had many other people walk into my consulting room, who take complete responsibility for their own health and seek advice to help them with their health-care specifics. They will look at the options, measure the advice, carefully consider their choices and ultimately do what they feel is best for them, even if that means going against the tide of popular opinion. They want to work in cooperation with the health-care practitioner. They demand to be treated as intelligent adults and do not respond well to a didactic approach.

Different Courses for Different Horses

When people are scared, which is understandable when they are dealing with certain health problems, they can easily regress to a child-like state. When in that state they might quickly hand over all choices and all responsibility to the 'parent-like' practitioner.

Ida was diagnosed with a chronic, slowly progressing form of heart failure. She bravely continued her life despite her illness and her needing to regularly attend her doctors and the hospital for her treatment. She was the most compliant patient on earth, never complaining and never questioning her health-care management. In fact she did not want to know any details of her illness and its management, only details of where and when she had to attend for her tests and treatment. She had no questions for her doctors and had utter trust in what they were doing. She would never entertain exploring other health-care approaches.

Ida had been raised in a family that would never even consider questioning those who they considered to be in authority. The 'they' always knew better and were beyond question. Ida never once discussed her prognosis, almost as though she had no right to enquire about her own illness. She felt it was not her responsibility to do so. She remained in that surrendered state until eventually she succumbed to her illness. That approach was, in its own way, perfect for her.

Angie consulted me for some hormonal problems and was found to have a number of other health concerns that required a series of investigations and various treatments. This was quite overwhelming for her initially as it was also at a time when she was trying to establish her business. When the shock of her medical concerns settled, and many of her health issues were attended to, she gained more control over the direction of her health and what management she did and did not want.

Angie had a very soft, gentle nature, yet I could see her strength come to the fore as she followed her own knowing regarding what she felt was best for her. During this time she appeared to gain a greater sense of self. She carefully listened to guidance yet maintained control of the direction of her health care. In her gentle way she demanded respect. She regained her health and vitality and went on to succeed in her business.

This is not to judge anyone's approach to seeking health care; and I am not suggesting, by the above examples, that one's approach will determine the outcome, as there are many factors at play. It really is a matter of 'different courses for different horses'. What will suit one might not necessarily suit another, as in all areas of life; and we can never really judge what one decides is best for them. However, both practitioner and patient should have the right to abide by methods and boundaries that are right for them and not continue a therapeutic relationship if their preferences are being transgressed.

Mistakes

'Let he who is perfect cast the first stone…'

We all make mistakes. How could we not? However, even deeming something a 'mistake' is a judgement. Is there really such a thing? Of course we need to learn from behaviours and actions that might have caused harm to self or others. This is a continuous life process. Remorse and guilt are sometimes very appropriate in the short term and it would be very concerning if one was not capable of feeling these emotions. When we allow ourselves to fully feel them and be guided by them in the moment, the less likely we will maintain them at an unconscious level, from which they will do more harm to our psycho-biological systems.

Everyone is choosing, in the moment, what they feel is best to do, or not do, given their life experience and their level of development and knowledge at the time. This is the case even if what they do is considered a crime. There are a million influences on a person's decision in the moment. We can never fully know what these influences are for ourselves, let alone another. Hindsight, however, might give us very different information. When we are living an *unconscious* life, we actually do not have free will and are responding to our *programming*, which includes a multitude of factors, including our priorities and beliefs. For the sake of ourselves, and humanity as a whole, it pays to get conscious.

It is very easy in hindsight to suggest that another action should have been taken. But you did not know *then* what you know *now*; even if *then* was only two hours ago. You would always have made the same choice. We are continually upgrading our knowledge by our experience and education. When practising medicine, we learn the most from our greatest mistakes. We never forget them and will never repeat them. We dread making mistakes as there is so much at stake and we just do not want to cause harm to another.

We are subject to a very punitive system – where we are expected to do all things perfectly all of the time. This is not possible for any human being, particularly when under (sometimes extreme) pressure. It is actually inhumane to expect so. And nobody, in his or her right mind, goes to work thinking: "What mistake can I make today?"

Maybe the bigger picture is that an individual attracted, or was scheduled to have, a certain experience, no matter what that might be, for their greatest learning and evolvement. This is a philosophical point of view but it makes as much rational sense to me as any other explanation of how life works. Who is the final arbitrator of what is 'right' or 'wrong' and what one should or should not have experienced? Who is the great 'they' who exerts this power and dominion over the majority? I believe we can only ever decide that for ourselves, not for any other, even though a consensus is sometimes beneficial for the majority.

Yes, of course we should aim for excellence in care with the highest standards being upheld and all reasonable measures taken to protect the public from malpractice. However, a punitive system forces many practitioners to operate from fear rather than common sense. Having to have perfect knowledge and do things perfectly at all times is way beyond what is reasonable, possible, and humane. In my profession we say that we are always learning. If we are always learning, then we never know it all; and we never will know it all as knowledge and experience is not finite and is ever-evolving. What was held sacrosanct at one point in time is often later decided to be incorrect.

As said, there are millions of influences impinging upon any decision one might make at any one time. There is obviously much commonality in what we experience, however, there is also much experience that each individual has that is unique to him or her. An individual's experience might be such that their decision would, by general consensus, be considered to be faulty. This would then mean that their wisdom and knowledge would need to be up-graded, and better by education than punishment.

Litigation!

Recently I read of a case where a doctor, a general medical practitioner, was sued for failing to refer his patient for bariatric surgery. The patient apparently suffered from diabetes and had a history of alcohol problems and had repeatedly failed to follow health-care advice. He apparently had previously been referred to a hospital diabetes clinic and to a hospital weight-control clinic – both of which, one would hope, would discuss weight loss and nutrition.

Now, one could argue that if bariatric surgery was always successful and safe, there might be an argument for proactively referring the patient. In my experience I have seen enough unsuccessful cases, and cases fraught with complications, that I believe one would have to very carefully consider the pros and cons of the procedure before persuading a patient to go down that path. Some people benefit greatly from this surgery, but it is not without risk.

Most people are very aware of the benefits of good nutrition and exercise but there is *not* a linear relationship between food intake and body weight. It is just not as simple as that as there are many subconscious influences at play regarding body weight; ideally these are addressed to help bring about a healthy outcome. Any surgery is dealing with the effects, not the *cause* of a condition.

So where does the responsibility start and end? Is it expected that health-care practitioners take their patients by the hand and lead them to their appointments and monitor their every move? We are not their parents. Where is personal responsibility in all of this?

Doctors have been sued for 'wrongful birth', meaning they have been held responsible for the unwanted birth of a child, and the *harm* inflicted on the parents by not having alerted the parents that the child might potentially have a serious genetic or chromosomal abnormality. Somehow the plaintiffs have no responsibility for the conception of their own child. It is the doctor's entire fault. The plaintiffs do not like the experience of having a child with a condition (which might actually have been their greatest blessing and greatest means of learning, if they chose to see it that way), therefore are 'harmed' by the situation – and somebody has to pay.

More so, a doctor can be sued for 'wrongful life', in which case the child sues the doctor – for their very existence. No wonder doctors have a reputation of playing God – because they are expected to! Nobody, no matter who they are or what they do, can have that much power over life, nor be given the burden of that much responsibility. Nature and life does not get it wrong – we do, by our attitudes, fuelled by our social conditioning toward what we experience. What message is this giving to the world? It just further fuels the victim/blame mentality that is already so entrenched and a scourge on our society.

Most doctors pay thousands of dollars annually for medical indemnity insurance. It is assumed we are likely to make a 'mistake' even before we start. Despite sacrificing countless evenings and weekends on various seminars, webinars and workshops (at our own considerable expense) to keep up-to-date, we are punished before we even don the stethoscope. This is considered entirely normal and expected. Well it is not normal, but entirely based on a misunderstanding of how life works.

I look forward to the day when the negative aspects of this system of litigation come crumbling down like the Berlin wall, whilst the positive aspects are maintained to reasonably protect the community against negligent malpractice.

There are myriad factors converging on why someone might experience certain things at certain times. To lay the blame on any one thing or one person is simplistic and based on a misconception. We cannot determine, nor control all of the many factors impinging on another's experience of life. We are conditioned to look for a scapegoat, someone to blame and point the finger at, and to absolve ourselves of all responsibility when we experience the unwanted. It is a way of avoiding what we personally feel at a deep level.

Who Plays God?

Our collective fear and denial of death has contributed to this punitive environment. It drives much of what we do in the medical arena. We have the belief that death is the ultimate tragedy, and avoidable. Do we really have an influence on the timing of someone else's death? Our belief-structure and medical system suggest that we do; after all that is what the practise of medicine is all about isn't it – to save lives?

Maybe being supported by good medical care were the circumstances that helped the patient survive when they had determined, at whatever level of their being, they were going to survive anyway; and maybe another person was going to die when they were going to die, despite all efforts to help them survive. Who really knows?

This is not at all to suggest that good medical care and all efforts to help a person to have a long, healthy life should not be exercised. I am just suggesting that we should not be expected to play God. Regarding the outcome of another, a lot of what happens is out of our hands. Ultimately, it is up to the individual and their personal connection to that creative intelligence. We just play our role in supporting the outcome they, at some level, might have already determined. We do not have as much power, regarding our effect on the outcome of others, as we might like to think!

'Rinchen'

Many years ago I sat by a child as he died. It was when I was working at a small hospital nestled in the foothills of the Western Himalaya in North India, above Dharamsala, the capital of Tibetans-in-exile. This hospital ran a tuberculosis-control program, as tuberculosis was very prevalent in Tibetans living in India. The hospital had a long tradition of Australian volunteer doctors and I was working there in that capacity.

Rinchen was a 10-year-old boy who lived at the 'Tibetan Children's Village' (TCV) in the foothills above Dharamsala. TCV was home to many Tibetan 'orphan' children, many of who were sent by their families in Tibet to live in a place that allowed cultural and religious freedoms.

With skinny limbs, a belly swollen with tuberculosis and a ready, cheeky smile, Rinchen was a regular at the TCV medical clinics we ran as an outreach service from Delek Hospital. He had disseminated tuberculosis and had not responded to the various anti-tuberculosis drugs that we had available. Even a stint at a larger, more sophisticated hospital in the south did not help him overcome his illness.

One cold, clear night he was rushed down the mountain from TCV to our little hospital. He had developed acute respiratory distress and was getting worse by the minute. On arrival, Rinchen was obviously very unwell, 'in extremis' (which was not uncommon in those parts, in those times, when people sometimes had to undertake a long journey before receiving medical care).

He was breathing as fast as his little body could manage, with every accessory muscle in use, and he was clearly tiring. Never complaining, he was totally absorbed by his frail body's efforts to survive. Auscultation revealed virtually no air entry to his lungs. A chest x-ray demonstrated more 'white-out' than aeration; and tests such as blood gases etc. were way beyond the diagnostic capabilities of the hospital at that time.

I was on duty, alone, apart from Tsering Dolma, a nurse, who was quietly attentive, efficient, knowing. She had seen it all before. Apart from the two of us there was nobody to consult or exchange ideas with. There was no lab running sophisticated tests, nor helicopter ambulance to take him to a tertiary hospital for specialist care.

Rinchen was given a cocktail of oxygen, antibiotics, diuretics, bronchodilators, steroids, medication to relieve his discomfort – and prayer. Rinchen did not respond to anything, his rapid breathing continuing like a train at full speed. It was a seemingly endless night. There were no heroics here. Rinchen slipped into unconsciousness and died as dawn was breaking.

The inevitable questions of 'What else could I have done to help this child survive or at least decrease his discomfort?' were buffered by the local community's quiet acceptance that it was just time for this little battler to move on. Always experience to be gained and lessons to be learnt, but not necessarily in the way we would choose.

No doctor goes to work thinking 'Whose death might I be contributing to today?' but I bet there is not one of us, who has worked long enough, who has not left a shift at some time thinking 'What else could I have done to give this person some relief or avert their death?' 'Might I have done something wrong, overlooked something, or made a 'mistake' that contributed to that person's outcome?' Who in this profession has not had some sleepless nights?

This is a heavy burden we often gloss over as part of the job. In my opinion, nobody should have to bear that much responsibility for another. Do our very best, yes, but with reasonable, common-sense understanding of how much influence we really do have regarding the outcome of another. Some of the outcomes are just going to be out of our hands, despite our best efforts.

Forgiveness

In my opinion, we forgive when we forgive and not a moment before. To force forgiveness just does not sit well with me, particularly if it is to gain some spiritual brownie points; and I believe that to force forgiveness too early, when we are not ready, and have not matured those emotions, can cause more harm than good.

To reach forgiveness we sometimes have to wade through those painful emotions such as anger, resentment and sadness that might stand in the way. Putting a veneer of 'forgiveness' on top, because we think we *should,* is a short-cut that does not work. The emotions and the related beliefs that stand in the way of true forgiveness need to be brought out of hiding, acknowledged, and dealt with. This is straightforward and easy for some, and more challenging for others.

Obviously forgiveness *is* the ultimate social, psychological and spiritual ideal for which to aim; but for some it might be a life's journey to get there. There (forgive me!) can be a certain spiritual 'political correctness' regarding forgiveness. Even the fact that we feel we need to forgive implies a sort of moral superiority. True forgiveness will be when the word loses its meaning and we see that there is actually *nothing to forgive.*

When we accept our own and the other's humanness, and see there is a bigger picture where we are all acting out our dramas through our own filters; where we all play a role in what circumstances we attract to ourselves – we are more likely to forgive self and others. True forgiveness is when the illusions are lifted.

This does not mean we put up with or condone actions that have harmed us, or others. Sometimes we have to make a firm stance against them. That might be part of our expression of self-love and the journey to feeling more empowered. However, it helps to also recognise that other people, and life circumstances, might be mirroring what we are holding in our own consciousness. Changing our experiences is mainly an internal job, with action inspired by alignment to a higher ideal for all.

We are continually learning from each other through our differences and issues. I remember a very successful person sharing that in his youth he had been drinking hard until one day when he saw an inebriated person behaving shamefully. At the moment of witnessing this he decided to give up drinking and change his life course. He posed the question: 'Was that person's purpose in life to teach others to *not* go down the same path as he had?' Others will teach us, by example, what to do and what *not* to do. We are not necessarily privy to the bigger picture, and we can never really judge. As is said, our greatest 'soul mate' might be our greatest enemy, for they will teach us the most.

To forgive, you have to decide that you want to do so and then intend that forgiveness will happen in the best and quickest way possible. It is a choice. Then see what transpires to bring this about. When you have really decided you want forgiveness to be the outcome you will be amazed at how life can coordinate events to culminate in you realising this state. You will know when you have truly forgiven and removed those illusions.

Emotions such as anger, resentment, bitterness and victimisation, that might oppose forgiveness, just do not feel good in the body. That is reason enough to transform them. This process might involve allowing ourselves to feel these emotions as they are moving through and out of our system. When I have kidded myself that I am justified in having these emotions, and therefore resist the release of them, my body will indicate that holding onto them is not in my (or anyone else's) best interests. Of course if we hold onto them long enough the body might then give us a stronger indication – and we sometimes call this illness.

You will never feel as liberated as when you *truly* forgive. That, of course, and maybe particularly, includes forgiveness of self.

From Trauma to Triumph

This discussion is in no way to minimise the marked traumas and injustices people can experience. They should be met with the greatest of understanding and compassion. However, we always have a choice as to how we respond to given circumstances, what we glean from those experiences and what we carry forth from them. We can feel great grief or betrayal at times but also have the overview that we are, at some level, responsible for how we choose to grow through all of our experiences.

When we are run by our unconscious programming, and related beliefs and defences, we do not even *realise* we have some choice regarding how we respond to our life circumstances. We often need appropriate education to upgrade our understandings, and ideally at an individual and societal level.

It is understood that some people experience hardships, tragedies and losses beyond normal human comprehension. They need to be met with the greatest of compassion and support. Sometimes the best we can do for them is to hold them in our hearts. We often just do not know why things happen as they do and why people might have to suffer so much. We will never fully understand another's life journey, though empathy arises when we experience some commonality. Therefore we can never really judge another, nor take on others' judgement of ourselves.

When people have experienced hardship and trauma, beyond that of normal human experience, the effects on them might never be fully understood by those who have not had similar experiences. The positive thinking brigade can seem very dismissive and even harsh towards those appealing for understanding of their situation. It is very easy for those who have been born into a feathered nest to give advice; but it might well fall on deaf ears if given from a lofty position of separation from 'heart-knowing' of others' plights.

It can be very invalidating and harmful to tell another to 'just get over it', particularly for those who experienced significant adverse early-life events, which can have such significant repercussions, and set the tone, for the rest of their lives. For people who have not experienced similar, in my opinion, they are just not qualified to give advice. The best teachers and mentors are those who have taken themselves through a journey that might resonate with that of their students. They can teach others how to best learn from their experiences and ultimately move on and let go of their past. They can demonstrate that it is indeed possible to fully heal from adversities.

Life can be hard and many, if not most people experience some significant difficulties during their lifetime. Everyone has a hero's story to tell and everyone needs another to 'bear witness' to their story. In fact, it is a great privilege to be in the position of being able to be present to others' life stories and experiences.

If people cannot recount their distress, if there is no verbal outlet, there is the risk of their emotional experiences adversely affecting their physical health. It is very appropriate that we voice our hurts, pains and sufferings to another. This is what, human to human, we can do for each other. However, it does pay to be discerning regarding with whom to share your story, and when the story is better left behind.

I do believe that people who have endured great hardships should be acknowledged and honoured. This helps us to recognise the strength of the human spirit, and helps us acknowledge that these individuals have helped humanity forge a better way. Many of our forebears suffered and sacrificed so that their descendants did not have to. We all have a related story in our family trees. Nothing that they experienced was in vain. It can be very dismissive to gloss over what people have experienced, out of our own ignorance and our attempts to be positive and upbeat.

A more metaphysical viewpoint is that one might experience challenges in the form of 'initiations' to quickly address aspects of their consciousness that are calling to be changed. This is for the sake of raising the vibration of their consciousness (from which everything else springs) to a level that is more aligned with love and wisdom, rather than fear and misconceptions. This is for the benefit of the individual and humanity as a whole.

We humans have done pain and struggle very well for millennia. Maybe we have now evolved to a point where there is an easier way. We have believed that hardship is our birthright, but hopefully we will evolve to a state where we see peace and bliss as our birthright. We have been programmed to believe that pain and struggle are beneficial and that we will be rewarded for sacrifice and martyrdom. I believed this for decades. In fact, I still have the tendency to think that I have to struggle and apply great effort if I am to achieve anything worthwhile. I am realising this is a good belief to *change.*

Sure we can learn and grow from our struggles and our manifold life experiences; a positive can always be gleaned from difficult experiences. However, we can experience joy and happiness and also grow through that. Part of the lesson from struggle and pain is to find ways to reduce or avoid struggle and pain, to forge a better way.

By recognising what we don't want, we can gain the impetus to turn this around to what we *do* want. It is about transmutation to a state *beyond* suffering. It is said that we are entering a more enlightened age where our consciousness will be elevated to a level where the hardships of our collective past will become a dim memory. We have done the hard yards. Time for more happiness, harmony and joy, I think!

The Meaning of Crisis

Sometimes 'crises' will steer you away from what is not working well in your life, to a situation that is ultimately more conducive to your happiness. You might fight tooth and nail to avoid upheaval in your life, but it is nature's way of putting you back on track to what is in your highest good. Serious illness is a crisis, as are accidents. Any significant change can feel like a crisis, even though change is inevitable. Upheaval will get your attention. It is life being on your side, though it sure does not feel like it at times. Of course you do not have to wait for a crisis to occur before you make positive changes in your life or attitudes.

The outcome of crises is to restore balance, to change old patterns that are actually not serving you well and that have been maintained out of habit. Crises shake up old, entrenched patterns and misconceptions. They are transformative and growth-enhancing, as they flush out stagnant attitudes and ways of being. They help us dismantle the illusions. We have been taught to view crises through the lens of the victim. Nobody wants a crisis to occur in his or her life and it is best to avoid them if you can. There are less traumatic and more elegant ways to embrace the changes that might be necessary for our growth.

Adrianna presented at a time when she was going through a crisis related to her work. She was in a position where she was worked to exhaustion, did not feel valued, and was generally treated poorly by her workplace. This was in addition to some ongoing family issues that demanded her time and energy. She was very experienced and good at her profession but felt she was being forced into an early retirement because of the level of stress she was experiencing.

When she presented to me she was clearly exhausted and depressed. We decided that it was best for her to have some time away from work to give her the space to address and recover from her stress and exhaustion. During this time she re-evaluated her position. She decided to not return to her workplace. Adrianna later found a much more suitable position where her skills and experience were acknowledged and where she was treated with respect.

During this transition she adopted a much healthier lifestyle, took some time to 'smell the roses' and was able to create a happier work/life balance for herself. Some counselling helped her to regain her sense of self and re-discover what she enjoyed. In the past she had loved acting and during this time joined a local amateur-theatre group, which has since become a significant and joyful part of her life.

Had Adrianna not experienced this crisis she might not have made the changes that brought about a much happier lifestyle and a more in-depth knowing and appreciation of herself and what she enjoys in life.

Alchemy

The concept of alchemy, the turning of base metal into gold, can be a metaphor for some aspects of health care and healing. Out of difficult experiences can arise qualities such as endurance, patience, resilience, understanding, empathy and wisdom. Our achievement-oriented, 'look at me' society does not necessarily give value to these qualities, as they are not adrenaline-fuelled and on show; however, though they often fly under the radar, they are the glue that holds humanity together.

The opposite of victimhood is looking back on all of your experiences and seeing them as perfect for having developed the wonderful qualities you now have. Many people, in hindsight, would not change a thing in their life, as they realise they have gained so much through all they have experienced, and have used their life experiences to elevate their consciousness to a higher level. To evolve, your consciousness needs something to work on.

Through all that we experience there is the potential for growth and the development of a better way. It pays to look for those gold nuggets. You will all have had experiences where, in retrospect, you might have considered that a situation, which was not appreciated at the time, was the best thing that ever happened to you. In hindsight we can glean the gifts.

Gratitude

It is said that gratitude is one of the highest vibration emotions and that those who practise gratitude and appreciation will attract to themselves more for which to be grateful.

Much can go awry with our bodies but much works very well most of the time. We can easily forget this. We have trillions of cells that are getting on with the job of keeping us on the planet.

Just the fact that our hearts tick away continuously in the background without any conscious thought at all is beyond amazing. It pays to tune into your body with gratitude, as the body will respond well to this attitude. Gratitude and appreciation are much higher on the Richter scale than fear and apathy, and thus they are more wellness-inducing.

You can apply gratitude to anything. Certainly to things you like and appreciate, but also to situations and things to which you might be more averse. It is not a matter of forcing the emotion but genuinely looking for aspects to appreciate. You might be grateful for a situation you did not enjoy because it taught you so much and propelled you into the direction of what you *do* like. There is always something to find if you choose.

I was very fortunate to have been brought up in a family that knew the body could heal from most things, and with as little interference as possible. I understood that the body knew what to do if we just let it get on with the job. Medical advice was sought infrequently, only when we knew it was really needed, rather than as a first-stop approach.

So I have learnt to be grateful for my body and trusting that it will do what it knows to do – sometimes with a little coaching from my mind! I expect my body will function well and heal most things. I am not pretending I have not had my physical challenges or that I won't have more. I know I will experience them if my consciousness needs to. However, I am grateful for this physical vehicle that has carried me through many adventures.

Some years ago I injured my right shoulder and as a result experienced excruciating pain. I knew I had done something significant to my shoulder and was also aware of the sorts of mind-body issues that might be related to this physical manifestation. Rightly or wrongly, I decided to not go down the track of MRIs, surgery, etc. (I am not suggesting that you do the same!). I did have a few sessions with a chiropractor and a kinesiologist and I am sure this helped.

The pain was more than I had ever experienced and, being right handed, was aggravated by any movement of my right arm. Analgesics did not even take the edge off so I abandoned them very quickly. The way I got through this was to focus on the parts of my body that were *not* in pain, intend that my body would heal as quickly as possible, and determine that any related emotional factors would be addressed and resolved. I was grateful for having learnt some tools I could use and for being given an opportunity to heal the deeper issues that underlie this experience.

The pain was marked for over two weeks and I was starting to wonder if I was ever going to be free of it. Being a mother with two young children at the time, I still had to attend to my day-to-day tasks. In fact, getting on with life was a welcome distraction from the discomfort. I *willed* my shoulder to heal.

When the condition was a little improved I gently resumed my work-outs at the gym. Now this might seem like a crazy thing to do (and I am *not* suggesting you do the same as I know my own body and can experiment with it. I cannot do that with yours). However, I knew that going to the gym was not going to be an issue and that actually it would enhance my healing. This is because the emotional component of my injury was not at all related to the gym environment and the gym reminded me of health and strength; and I could put more emphasis on the parts of my body that were working well. From then my recovery was rapid.

My father, when aged 88, fractured his right knee-cap and bones in his left elbow. This occurred when he was in the city on a rainy day and slipped on a curb when standing back to let someone pass on the footpath. After falling he got himself up and proceeded to catch the tram to meet his friend for lunch as had been arranged. When he met his friend it was then decided that they had better call an ambulance.

At the hospital the fractures were diagnosed and he proceeded to have surgery on his elbow. Following a few days in hospital he had a short stint in a rehabilitation centre. Despite some dour predictions regarding his recovery from those around him, he healed more quickly than would be expected for someone a third of his age.

During this process I could sense that he was completely relaxed and surrendered to the situation whilst fully expecting that his body would heal. Which it did. He did not even consider that it would not. Since then, some years later, I have never once heard him complain of any residual pain, disability or restriction related to the accident. For me, this was a glowing example of the potential to recover when one is *grateful* for their body's capacity to heal, and *expects* that it will get on and do so.

Gratitude is the opposite of victimhood and will attract to us more to be grateful for. The practise of gratitude can be a daily practise that will hold you in very good stead. Don't force it. Find things you are genuinely grateful for and start with the small stuff. This can be related to health or life in general. If you have an ache in your elbow, be grateful your big toe feels fine, and be grateful your body is giving you a message.

Send appreciation to your body as it will much better respond to this energy than to the energy of fear or rejection. This is not 'head in the sand' as you know it is appropriate to get professional help with any health concerns you might have. Trusting in your own body's capacity to heal does not preclude seeking health care when needed. If experiencing health concerns, trust that your body will heal in the best and easiest way, and this might include some professional help.

Do You Choose to Remain a Victim or a Master of Your Own Health?

Do you prefer to believe your health and wellbeing are due to genetics, fate, or good or bad luck; or that you have some conscious control of your experiences, or at least of your reaction to them? Do you choose to remain a victim or a master of your own health? You will not lapse into victimhood if you understand that you grow through your experiences, regardless of what they might be, and can, at least in part, determine the direction of your own life, including your health.

To bring about real change, one needs to become aware of, and question, the conditioning and programming one has bought into. You will not experience what you do not believe, and we are all subject to many compelling beliefs regarding illness outcome. We need to be educated otherwise. It is time to upgrade our collective beliefs.

A certain amount of inertia might need to be overcome for one to undertake the journey of inner exploration and change. This can be very difficult if one is a long way down the illness trail and has little energy with which to engage such things, and especially if they are not familiar with these concepts. However, we know people can and do turn things around quickly, even if very unwell, if they have the determination and choose to do so. We all know of people who defy all odds. It is helpful to seek out their stories for inspiration.

Not everyone wants to do the 'hard yards' and take on the task of exploring their inner dimensions, especially when they are feeling unwell, frightened or overwhelmed. Health-care practitioners need to respect individuals' choices and work with *their* reality whilst not disrespecting their own understandings.

Of course, in addition to doing the inner work (i.e. addressing consciousness-related factors), one needs to support the body as best they can. Appropriate health-care advice on physical aspects, such as diet, medications, herbs, etc. should be sought and given. That goes without saying. Working with mind and body are not mutually exclusive, as it is all connected. It is a matter of 'working from the inside out and the outside in'. Holistic health care encompasses the whole.

Conclusion

We all feel victimised by life at times. It is part of the human experience. The journey is from victimhood to empowerment. It is about transitioning from helplessness and blame to self-responsibility and inner strength. You might have heard the term 'to make lemonade out of lemons'. If you suffer an adversity why not milk it for all that you can? Why not gain the utmost you can from it? It helps to see adversities as *opportunities,* as so much learning and positive change can result from them. It is helpful to have role models and mentors who have knowledge of the journey at a personal, experiential level, and who know how to successfully manoeuvre through it. Maybe you will be that role model for others.

At all times you need to be true to what you *really* feel. Sometimes we just feel life has thrown us a curve ball that defies all understanding of why it might have happened. Acknowledging and allowing those emotions, when true and appropriate, is very different to maintaining them so that they become a way of being. It is normal and healthy that you let those emotions come to the fore and at the level that they are honestly felt. Paradoxically, when you allow yourself to feel your pure emotions instead of holding onto the related 'story', you are much less likely to lapse into victimhood, blame and resentment.

It is said that life, as we experience it, is a mirror to what we hold in consciousness. Though we cannot directly control other people – nor should we – we can control what we invite into our arena. As said, we are not necessarily privy to the deeper workings of our consciousness and what we might have chosen to experience to accelerate our growth. If you never had a challenge, problem or adversity, likely you would vegetate, as there would be no reason to extend yourself, grow and evolve. Likely you would not be here in this vast learning field of life on Earth.

You learn and grow the most when you are stretched a little; when you have to push beyond what you already knew. You will not grow if you do not reach beyond self-imposed or conditioned limitations. Sometimes your greatest adversaries and your most difficult experiences are your greatest gifts – if you decide to grow through them, rather than be victimised by them.

As previously stated, the basic question is: "Is life on your side and all that you experience is for your growth and development?" or "Is life not supporting you and you have to struggle, fight or manipulate to survive?" You choose. Consider that 'Life' is conspiring to use whatever it takes for you to reach your greatest growth and highest potential. What if all you have experienced is to refine your wisdom, and your intent of what you really do want to experience in life, so that the suffering dissipates to allow joy?

End of Chapter Points

- *Everyone will feel victimised at times. It is an archetypal pattern we are all working through.*

- *Adverse early-life experiences might set up a pattern of making one feel victimised by life.*

- *Resentment and blame are the by-products of feeling victimised.*

- *It can be very easy to feel victimised by your health challenges. It helps to see them as opportunities for growth, rather than cause for victimisation.*

- *Any emotions, related to feeling victimised, are better met with compassion rather than judgement.*

- *When you allow yourself to honestly feel those emotions, and then let them go, you are less likely to carry them as victimisation.*

- *When we understand that we all, at some level of our being, attract to us what we experience, we will feel less victimised by life and more motivated to make positive changes.*

- *The more you relate your happiness to factors external to yourself, the more vulnerable you are to feeling victimised by life. You will be empowered when you realise that happiness is an inside job.*

- *The journey is from victimhood to empowerment. This can be a life-long journey with many helpful learning steps along the way.*

- *Empowerment equates to taking responsibility for yourself and your life as best you can.*

- *Healthy boundaries and good self-care enhance personal empowerment.*

- *When you see that life is really on your side, and that all that you experience is for your growth and the evolvement of your wisdom, you will feel less victimised. In fact, you might even feel grateful.*

- *What makes you feel the most victimised can sometimes be what most puts you onto the path to personal empowerment.*

Chapter 7

The Meaning of Illness

"We are not so much meant to heal our illnesses as they are meant to heal us."

CARL JUNG
(1875-1961, SWISS PSYCHIATRIST)

I do not know why people get sick. Yes, I might know at a biochemical and physiological level, and even at an emotional and energy level; however, I do not know of all the mysteries that underpin the vagaries of our human experience, including the experience of illness. There might always be some mystery that no amount of dissecting will reveal. I like to think everything happens for a reason and that ultimately nature, and universal intelligence, is on our side. I know this can sound very glib to those who are undergoing significant health challenges and considerable suffering. But what is the best alternative view? I am open to suggestion.

Why do we not just take for granted that our bodies will be reliable vehicles through which we experience this life journey? Why should 'health' even exist as separate category in our human lives? Is there a basic design fault underlying why our bodies can experience so much dysfunction? Has life just got it wrong? Or are our bodies the reliable indicators of what we hold in mind/consciousness, providing us with feedback at every moment? Are our bodies the means through which we learn? Maybe the experience of illness is our greatest means of learning and growth.

We are not necessarily privy to the deeper workings of our consciousness and to why we experience certain life situations, including health challenges. Much happens at a deeply unconscious level that our intellects might struggle to understand. It seems that consciousness gets what consciousness needs for its expansion and growth, and this might include the experience of illness. We just do not necessarily applaud the circumstances.

Our ego-personalities might try to make very different choices to those of our inner selves; yet, I believe, our inner selves eventually win. Illness, as well as other life challenges and adversities, makes us enter more into ourselves to address what we have been holding in those deeper levels of consciousness. If significant, this can be a 'dark night of the soul', from which we can eventually arise, as though from the ashes.

I remember a person advising me, during one of my times of distress, to just keep my personality out of it and let my soul get on with the job. Well, easier said than done! I was little comforted by those words, as my personality is the aspect I identify with, and the aspect that seems to be doing most of the experiencing on this life journey. And it can certainly be a stubborn little aspect that thinks it knows best and can be full of resistance to any indications from its inner, wiser counterpart.

As I am sitting here writing this (maybe I should be resting!) my body is permeated with the 'flu virus. I had taken pride in the fact that I had maintained robust health and not experienced even a sniffle throughout winter – until the last few days of winter. Then suddenly I was struck down. How could I go, in a matter of hours, from seemingly perfect health to an aching, mucous-dripping, coughing body, whose immune system seemed like it had chucked in the towel? Utterly inconvenient! So much to do! And there lies the problem. As I had over-committed and congested my mind with too many projects and too much study, I had become overwhelmed and had let stress mount. I put out a clear vibration for the virus to home in on. Perfect match!

My mind-body in its wisdom decided to withdraw from the pressures and slow down, and created the means to bring this about, i.e. the 'flu. A holiday might have been better but that was not on the agenda, as my personality had wanted to forge on regardless. The lesson? Maybe to not over-commit in the future and realise that like all humans there is just so much I can do before tipping the scales; and that I need a healthy, balanced lifestyle with adequate rest and recreation. Even that it is okay to have rest and recreation.

More so, if what was driving me was fear and ego, and based on trying to bolster my sense of self-worth and 'survive', rather than being led by heart-driven motivations – that is surely a recipe for stopping me in my tracks.

Much of what we treat as a dysfunction might actually be a compensation, an attempt of the mind-body to survive. For example, many of the symptoms of influenza are to temporarily slow us down, to force us to withdraw for a time when we have ignored the mental and emotional cues; our unwitting way of removing ourselves from the challenges of life for a while.

When we only prop ourselves up with various 'treatments' and don't address the underlying dysfunction we might get a louder message further down the track. Our physical bodies give us the messages we fail to heed at the mental, emotional and spiritual levels. Sometimes it is a simple message, or it can be an obvious wake-up call. It helps to view all of our experiences (including our health challenges) as worthwhile, the opportunity for learning, and part of our rich life journey.

Admittedly this can be difficult when we are in the midst of illness and feeling vulnerable, frightened, weak and unwell. At these times we might have to surrender to what we are experiencing whilst taking the very best care of ourselves and accepting good care from others. The insights might gently unfold as we tend to our health and hold the image of the best of outcomes for ourselves.

Gifts in Disguise

I have heard people say that they were 'given' an illness. Do they believe they were given an illness as a challenge, or maybe even as a punishment by some higher intelligence? Are we *given* an illness, or do we *create* an illness; or maybe attract an illness by the dominant vibration of the thoughts and emotions we emanate? Or do we at some level, *choose* an illness as a means of speeding up our learning and growth? Or is it that wake-up call? Maybe our bodies are the perfect means by which we can become aware when something is off track and when a higher learning is being called for.

I will hold to the belief that we inevitably grow through all of our experiences, and maybe particularly our physical challenges. I believe our ultimate aim is to evolve our consciousness and that everything else is secondary, but inextricably linked, to that. It sometimes takes circumstances beyond the ordinary to accelerate the growth of an individual, as well as that of a group; health challenges might be the perfect opportunity to motivate us to really address what needs to be changed in our minds and our lives. What goes on with our physicality gets our attention.

We are generally trained to gauge life's events and experiences by whether they bring us pain or pleasure. We are attracted to what we believe might give us pleasure and repelled by what we believe might induce pain. That seems like a normal, reasonable approach to life. However, it also pays to glean what we can from experiences we might not enjoy nor consciously choose.

We all know we are just a little wiser when we have overcome something; and even when we couldn't overcome it and had no choice but to surrender to it. Maybe an individual's experience of illness was for his or her learning of self at a deeper level. It might be just what one needed to change patterns that did not serve him or her well. It might be when the body says "enough!"

Maybe the illness experienced was always going to be, scheduled to fast-track one's growth, and circumstances complied to bring it about. Maybe one's inner being 'took it on' courageously for maximum growth and evolvement of themselves and others. Who knows?

We are not accustomed to looking at the positive side of health challenges. We all know of individuals, if not ourselves, who re-evaluated their lives and patterns, and whose strengths came to the fore because of the experience of illness. We are aware of those who conduct their healing journeys with amazing grace and courage, having an inspiring influence on those around them.

We are not isolated beings and we inevitably affect those around us, albeit often unwittingly. We are all, at some level, connected. Sometimes the lesson of our experience is not primarily for ourselves but for those around us who are observing. Inevitably, what we feel happens just within the confines of our own minds and bodies will reverberate out to affect others and *all of life*. This adds to the many ways in which we influence each other and how we all contribute to the collective. Our 'stuff' is not necessarily just our stuff; however, what we do with it is up to us individually.

I have the highest respect for people who have endured a host of adversities, including illness, physical or emotional trauma, and loss of loved ones. I particularly pay homage to them when they have turned their experiences around and gleaned some gifts, difficult though that might have been; and when they have shared their wisdom with others.

Many people, due to experiencing considerable challenges, go on to create much more fulfilling, happy, and heart-aligned lives for themselves. They are a shining inspiration for the rest of us, and very much teach by their example. These people demonstrate the strength of the human spirit and, particularly, that they are greater than their circumstances.

Having more control and choice regarding the outcome of our health and lives does require changing the beliefs that suggest that we do not. It involves knowing ourselves at a deeper level, and being aware of the many influences on us. We can also be comforted by knowing that, despite what we might decide to do or not do regarding our health or any other aspect of our lives, life will be teaching us regardless.

As previously mentioned, changing beliefs and upsetting the status quo is often met with much resistance, and it does take effort, determination and will. It suits some people very well to remain miserable if they can avoid risking change and looking at those aspects of themselves they have denied or suppressed. There are no rights and wrongs here. Everyone is entitled to do what they feel is right for them – and will get the perfect feedback regarding their choices.

It is helpful to be reminded we can also learn and grow through less traumatic ways, particularly if we have learnt to tune into ourselves and pay attention to those inner signals before they become an illness manifestation. It is very encouraging that we *do* appear to be evolving to a state where we have more conscious choice regarding the outcome of our health and our lives in general. We are unravelling the programming and conditioning that had encouraged us to feel helpless and victimised by our own health challenges and life in general.

We have done enough suffering already, don't you think? Maybe it is now time to grow through joy. Though it seems like a stretch at this point, maybe illness and disease will eventually fade away as it will no longer be a necessary means for our growth. This might do me out of a job, but I am all for that!

'Fix it' versus 'Heal It'

As Dr Albert Schweitzer (and Hippocrates before him) said, *"It is more important for the doctor to know the patient who has the disease than to know the disease that has the patient."*

The 'fix it' approach to health care, though appropriate and lifesaving at times, runs the risk of forgetting the person behind the condition, the history behind the person, and the messages our bodies are trying to give us. For example, when assessing one for heart disease we are very particular, even obsessive, about checking cholesterol levels and so on; but how often do we put importance upon that particular individual's life story? How often do we focus on what affected his or her *heart?*

How often do you try to 'fix' your body like it is a machine, rather than delve into the currents of disturbance lying at a level deeper to that of the physical effects? When we treat only the symptoms it is like taking the battery out of the alarm. That temporary annoyance will go away but the underlying dysfunction will continue unabated, potentially causing much more harm.

Healing involves perceiving some *meaning* behind the illness rather than seeing it as bad luck, or an affliction one has to be rid of. Some might even say the word 'healing' is based on a misunderstanding that something was 'wrong' in the first place, and that the term is still putting our focus on the problem rather than on wellness.

The need for healing presumes something is wrong and therefore needs to be 'fixed'. Some might argue there is absolutely nothing to fix or heal, that it is all playing out just as it should, with people learning precisely what they need to learn from the exact circumstances they are experiencing at that time. This is based on the understanding that universal intelligence makes no mistakes; and, as part of universal intelligence, nor do we. Nature does not get it wrong. We are just good at misinterpreting it!

When you are 'fighting' an illness what are you fighting but some aspects of *yourself!* That is you working against you. When we fight a disease we should be fighting the unresolved hurts, and related misunderstandings and misconceptions about life that gave rise to the disease in the first place; not the disease itself as that is just an indicator of a deeper unrest.

Insight, understanding and integration of relevant antecedent factors, as well as supporting the body as best one can, might be a better approach. We need to work *with* ourselves not against ourselves. A strong, steady determination to heal will put one in a better position than taking the fighting stance. However, it is not yet in the collective understanding, including our health-care system, to approach health care in this manner.

I shudder when I hear media campaigns promoting the 'fighting' stance against illness. These are often, though not always, directed against cancer. I do understand they are well-meaning and might make people feel more empowered; and this is a long way better than apathy, resignation and despair. However, I do believe we are putting our energies in the wrong direction. Where we put our focus, our reality will follow. We are inadvertently affirming our belief in our capacity for illness, and particularly our capacity to be victimised by illness.

As long as we continue to only look externally for the cause and take the 'fighting' stance, we might well be met with disappointment, despite the efforts applied. When we start looking for consciousness-related causes of illness rather than 'cures', we will start to get somewhere. When we are fighting the physical manifestations, we are fighting the *effects* rather than the cause.

Our un-wellness indicates there is something to address at a level beyond the physical. If we treat only the symptoms, the underlying imbalance, whether it is nutritional, environmental, mental, emotional, or spiritual – will manifest in the same or another way at another time. And further layers of compensation will be added to the dysfunction.

Even if we are suffering from a viral or bacterial infection, our susceptibility to the infection, and to how it might progress, is related to our own vibrational energy at that time. Our vibrational energy, what we are emanating from our being, is related to the thought-patterns, beliefs and the associated emotions we might be harbouring. Don't blame the messenger!

It is easy to forget the mind-body's wisdom and the messages it is trying to tell us. The body knows before the intellect does and we would be well advised to tune in. We rarely ask, "What is this symptom or illness trying to tell me?" We are just not trained to do this. This approach has not yet filtered into the collective.

I have certainly seen patients who have had persisting and annoying symptoms that have clearly been trying to get their attention. Often these symptoms defy conventional 'cures' and, understandably, often the patients get very frustrated about this. The physicality has so got their attention they do not necessarily appreciate exploring other domains, and often object to any suggestion that their minds might be involved. In fact, I have had patients leave my consulting room screaming abuse when I have dared to venture there. Talk of the mind-body connection can seem like insult and sheer madness to some people.

Particularly for chronic conditions that do not fit the 'medical model' and for which there are no proven effective treatments; attempting to treat only the symptoms is very often lengthy, costly, frustrating and inadequate. There must be another approach. The physical is the last place where a deeper dysfunction manifests. Even with apparent 'acute' conditions, the imbalance has been under the surface for some time. The energy of an unresolved emotion, or thought-pattern gone amiss, will be compensated for until it needs to find an outlet and this is often in physical form.

If we get a quick fix (though obviously this has its place) there is less incentive for us to make the lifestyle changes and do the inner work to help resolve the problem. It is easier to go on a cholesterol-reducing medication than change one's diet! In my opinion passive healing, without the client having to make any changes within themselves, will go only so far. We do not really have to exercise our self-examination muscle if it is all given to us from external to ourselves. We do not have to do the work. Very convenient for some!

Obviously it is appropriate at times to focus mainly on the physical aspects of an illness. Common sense does have to prevail. If one presents with a heart attack or acute appendicitis it is not necessarily a good time to go and process their childhood! Or if one has a sore throat, an in-depth mind-body analysis might not be appreciated. And at certain phases of an illness, one simply might not have the energy or determination to do the inner work – or choose not to. At those times they might be in a position of only being able to receive care from others. As said, there are no rights or wrongs here.

The out-dated paradigm of healing as 'fixing' is still dominant in our collective consciousness and it might take some time for this to change. The difference between 'treating' and 'healing' is that the latter is dealing with the cause of the condition within, rather than just the removal of symptoms. For true healing to occur, something must change within.

Healing and transformation are different concepts to fixing and treating. Implicit in the concept of 'fixing' is judgement that something is wrong, not up to par, not normal, whereas 'healing' is aimed at restoring one to wholeness. Healing involves integration rather than just removing or adding bits. The health-care practitioner facilitates the healing process in the client, but does not do the healing, which is an internal job. Willingness on the part of the client is a necessary factor. The client must take responsibility for implementing any changes that might be necessary.

One can never 'fix' another, even though it is still the prevailing health-care model. How could we? Who are we to do so? How, as individuals, do we know of the intricacies of another human being's mind/body and soul? Even to decide someone needs healing is a misconception we have all bought into. Maybe what they are experiencing is just perfect for their growth at this time. Who are we to say? Sure, we do the best we can to help another, given the system as it is and the limitations of what we know; but human-to-human, we cannot 'fix' another.

Ultimately there really is nothing to heal and it is all unfolding perfectly with each individual learning exactly what they need to by their circumstances and experiences. Part of that learning is to propel us to change what is not working for us. Collectively, however, we are a long way from believing this, and it is in our human nature to do what we can to aid another – and of course we should. However, fixing someone versus aiding someone to *transform* are two very different mind-sets resulting in two very different outcomes.

Resistance versus Flow

When we surrender to the wisdom of our bodies, including the manifestation of illness, we are in a better position to relinquish the resistance that can work against us and impede the learning inherent in the experience of illness. Resistance equates to contraction, which blocks the flow of life's energies.

I have heard spiritual masters say, "Do not resist anything"; which basically means trust life and all that it entails and trust our capacity to deal with it and grow through it. Universal Consciousness knows – but do we trust it?

Humanity has evolved to a point where we do have more conscious choice regarding the outworking of our lives; where we are undoing much of our programming that has kept us ignorant and entrapped into servitude to certain belief-patterns and ways of being. 'Resist nothing', yet apply more intention and choice. Accept what is, as it is, and when it is – and then choose to change it as you would like. The paradox is that the point of change is when we accept what is. It is a matter of reconciling acceptance of what is with a determination to evolve to a better way.

'Resist nothing' also means accepting our resistance, as that can be the truth of the moment. Breathe into it; acknowledge it; feel it – and then decide whether it is in your best interests to maintain it. What you resist, you suppress. It is all about awareness and getting to know yourself at an intimate level.

'What we resist persists and intensifies.' Resistance is not the answer and never has been. When I have the 'flu, the more I resist it, the more it remains entrenched. When I surrender to it (which is not the same as resignation), the more likely it will take its natural course and provide me with its inherent lessons. I am not suggesting people do not treat what needs to be treated. One can surrender to something and treat/heal it at the same time. We can be aware there is a 'bigger picture' whilst also attending to the details. Surrender is a subtle yet very different energy to that of resignation, and the opposite of resistance.

'Going with the flow' is accepting what is, when it is, as it is – maybe, particularly accepting ourselves, with all our good points and foibles. This is not the same as complacency, but an acceptance of what is in the moment, including its lessons *and* need for adjustments. We will be more accepting of the moment when we bring our presence and non-judgemental awareness to it. When you are accepting of and aligned with the natural flow of life, this will reflect positively in how your body functions.

When dealing with illness, it is beneficial to be surrendered to the process whilst at the same time doing what you can to heal (I do realise this is easier said than done!). Another paradox. When we grasp, strain, resist and fight, we are inadvertently maintaining what we are resisting. Behind any desperate approach is the dominant fear that what we want will not happen. A calm determination is a more helpful quality. We will heal when we *trust* and expect that we can.

Regarding the emotions you might experience during illness, being present with what you genuinely feel, rather than forcing yourself to be 'positive', will help bring to the surface and dissipate what might have contributed to the illness-causation in the first place. Healing at some level is inherent in the illness experience, if we allow it.

Paradoxically, when you accept what is as it is, you can then exercise your right to have priorities and preferences according to your genuine wants and needs. When you align with that universal intelligence and the flow of life, and release your resistance to what is in the moment, you will have an easier ride through life.

Going with the flow is also accepting ourselves as we are and the human condition as it is. Our humanness experiences 'blocks' at times, does not always act on what we intuitively know is for our highest good, and sometimes makes some foolish mistakes. Well at least mine does! Thank God, life will give us some reminders to keep us humble and get back on track; and thankfully life has a sense of humour!

The Healing Journey

We carry our past, particularly the unresolved, unintegrated aspects of our experience, in our bodies. I have seen countless people who believe they are over their past, and that they have no significant psychosocial factors to address, while their bodies tell me a very different story. I often hear them say they have had some counselling to deal with the past and what they have lived through is no longer significant. Consciously, they are often unaware of what they are still harbouring in their *subconscious* minds – and thus their bodies.

There are certain patterns of illness/dysfunction and clusters of physical disorders that appear to correlate with unresolved, and often deeply unconscious, early-life adverse experiences. We carry our interpretation of our past in our bodies by maintaining, in the now, thought-patterns and beliefs built upon what was formulated in those early years. This is where the real problem is.

These clusters of medical conditions might be called 'Functional Somatic Syndromes' and include conditions such as fibromyalgia syndrome, chronic fatigue syndrome, irritable bowel syndrome, certain autoimmune conditions, multiple food sensitivities and many others. (This is a generalisation and there are always exceptions to the rule.) These conditions usually have a multitude of symptoms, share much commonality of symptoms and are associated with significant debility. There is no denying they are real.

The symptoms might persist for years, if not decades. There might be some association with certain nutrient deficiencies, toxins and pathogenic organisms, but the link is often less than clear. There is rarely, if ever, a single defining symptom or pathology test or simple reliable treatment. Very challenging for client and practitioner alike! Of course the clients are frustrated and want to feel better and want to find that special key, whether it be a test result or therapy, which will help them. It rarely happens that way.

I do need to emphasise that when I refer to 'functional illnesses', or even 'psychosomatic' illnesses, it is not saying these illnesses are: "all in the head". The physical manifestations are very real; and, in my opinion, mind and body work together for every illness, for *everyone*. It is the chronicity of these illnesses that is so pertinent.

It is interesting that illness trends come and go. Of course this has much to do with public-health measures such as sanitation and vaccination; however, certain illnesses are more socially acceptable, and might I say 'popular', at different times in our history. And, to have a physical illness is often more socially acceptable than having unresolved childhood experiences, or difficulties with emotionally coping with the demands of life.

The sufferers are usually relieved if they do get a set diagnosis, some definition of their un-wellness. They very often want validation of their suffering and disability. They often go from practitioner to practitioner and spend a fortune on obscure tests to find obscure diagnoses, and elaborate therapies in an attempt to feel normal and engage life again. It is very easy for these people to feel victimised by the health-care system and life in general.

In my area, Lyme disease is a disease that is currently receiving a lot of focus. Well known in other parts of the world, it has been relatively recently recognised in this part of the world; and is *not* recognised by certain sectors of the medical fraternity. There is no doubt the disease is real and is associated with certain bacteria of the borrelia type and others, which are usually transmitted via a tick bite.

However, one wonders why *this* disease, and why *now*, and what might be the personal and collective mind-body associations that underlie it. Are the bacteria the sole causative agents, and it is just chance and bad luck regarding who is subject to this disease? Or, might there be broader issues at play? Do infectious agents *cause* diseases, or are they present as secondary agents *in response* to the milieu of the sufferer's mind and body? Do bacteria and viruses, as opportunists, hone in on a vibration already in place, or maybe even in an attempt to heal the underlying condition?

I suspect that when one is very much focussed on the physical aspects of what they are experiencing, they have suppressed the related emotional factors – past and present. The more one is removed from the mind/emotional causes of illness, the more they will have, and be focussed on, the physical manifestations. Classically this is what 'somatisation' means.

Body symptoms are a great distractor from what is really going on at a mind/emotional, and even spiritual, level. This really is an area of medicine where a holistic approach will help. Often these people stay on the illness journey for many years, but sometimes they ultimately heal themselves when given appropriate support and care. This truly can be a 'hero's journey' on many levels.

I suspect that many of the sufferers have unresolved, unintegrated early-life experiences from which thought-patterns, beliefs and defences are maintained, making the body so susceptible to these illness patterns. These people are often aware of having had trauma in their early lives but often gloss over it as insignificant and unrelated to their current health status.

When we do not engage and accept our experiences as they happen, learn the lessons/wisdoms inherent in them, and then relegate that experience to the past, we will carry them in our bodies. Deep emotional pain and difficult or challenging life experiences might have absolutely no adverse effect on our bodies if we fully deal with them at the time. It is much more of a concern if we suppress/repress our experiences, and unwittingly draw all sorts of beliefs and conclusions about life from them. Our physiology will indeed be adversely affected, as it follows suit from our thought-patterns, most of which are unconscious.

Of course we all suppress and repress at times, especially when we are young and do not have the ego strength, and often not the support, to fully deal with our experiences at the time they occur. Some of the experiences that potentially most adversely affect us, psychologically and physically, were experienced when we were very young, and even pre-verbal. Some might suggest, and I agree, that even what we experienced at our time of conception, during our time in-utero and at our time of birth can have the most potent influence on our later life. Though our brains were not fully developed, we still had an energy field at those early stages.

What we experienced might well have been neglect rather than trauma; and often what seem, in retrospect, like minor events. It is our *interpretation* of those experiences that counts. There often is no concrete memory to retrieve, nor language to rationalise it, but rather a pervasive feeling-sense that hovers in the background of awareness. Sometimes we just do not know what it is we are meant to be over. I doubt there is anyone on the planet who has not had some sort of early life trauma, but obviously some more than others.

Many would argue that it is never useful to go into one's past as it will be re-traumatising the client and putting the focus on the problem rather than on the solution. That can definitely be the case, and short medical consultations, and our health-care structure in general, do not usually allow this anyway. However, it depends on the intent. If the intent is to gain insight and integrate past experiences, so as to diminish their persisting ill effects, it is helpful. If it is to hang out in 'woundedness' and victimhood, and if it re-traumatises, obviously it is not.

As said it is not the experiences per se that is the problem but rather the *meaning* put on them, and what was derived from them that can so affect thinking patterns and thus later health. The defence mechanisms that we put in place in response to our perceptions of our life experiences can shut down the natural flow of energy and thus impede the natural functioning of our bodies.

It seems unfair, right, that the scene is often set when we are young, helpless and vulnerable? However, consciousness has no age, nor set time-line, and ultimately all is to heal our deeply-held distortions and misunderstandings about life. At some level, consciousness has a choice, no matter the age or state of the individual; and perhaps consciousness chooses to have certain experiences to heal at a level much deeper than our personality or the face that we present to the world.

I don't like to think it is just bad luck or fate, but rather a very clever ploy of consciousness (universal and personal alike) to realise and evolve aspects of itself through experiences in this physical reality. Some would suggest the whole object of life is for consciousness to expand through its experience of the many facets of itself. Obviously these views are open to conjecture.

Maybe we learn the most through contrast. By experiencing what we don't want we have more appreciation of, and determination to realise, what we *do* want. Held within ill-health is the potential for sublime health. Held within powerlessness and victimisation is the empowered state. Held within neglect and abandonment is inclusion and unconditional love.

We just have to put our sight on what we *do* want rather than maintaining the focus on what we no longer want to experience. What is the point in hanging around in pain? Illnesses and diagnoses, particularly, can be so compelling and can so take our focus that some effort needs to be exerted to counter this and steer in a different direction. At some point we have to have a clear intent to heal and it helps to call on the grace of a higher intelligence to assist us with this.

We forget that the body is always trying to keep us safe, and that nature does not get it wrong. The body is always doing its job, one way or another, even though it sometimes seems that it is failing us. Our bodies are always responding to the dictates of the mind. It is not our bodies that are failing us, but we who are failing our bodies.

Nature's Way

In the clinic's tea-room a group of young nurses were chatting on their break, discussing childbirth. They were projecting to their own future experience of childbirth. One young woman queried why anyone would not use pain-killers when they are available. To her and her friends it was incredulous that anyone in their right mind would not avail themselves to analgesia – as though it was the most natural thing in the world to do. To me it was incredulous that many, if not most, people consider that falsely taking away all pain and sensation is the norm.

My comment that it is good to be *present* during childbirth, and that the experience of pain is actually a culturally conditioned expectation, was met with blank stares and eye rolling. Possibly I was being a little self-righteous because at their age I would have had exactly the same opinion as them, and everyone has the right to choose what they feel is best for them. And whatever we do choose is perfect, as we will learn one way or another from those choices.

We do not live in a society that values wisdom and reflection, but rather seeks a rapid, mechanistic approach to our problems and this is reflected in our health care. We do not tolerate the smallest pains and discomfort without seeking some immediate relief. This applies as much, if not more, to emotional pain as to physical pain. We so quickly seek the little white pill that will take it all away. This has become a knee-jerk reaction, a conditioned response to any discomfort – and a righteous expectation.

All too often grief is medicated, not allowing one to go through its natural process until its acceptance and resolution. Often healing comes from facing the pain of the wound, whether it is physical or emotional, from staying *present* with the pain until it resolves. What if feeling sad, vulnerable or in grief is what you have to experience and work through in order to gain the wisdom from that experience, rather than medicate it away?

When fully present we will glean the lessons inherent in the experience, and then be more able to make choices to change what we might want to change as a result. Life has a way of making us revisit emotions we think we have successfully suppressed or skirted around. Suppression and denial have never served us well; however, it is still our tendency to seek comfort rather than growth. We have been trained to seek the easy way out rather than develop resilience.

Good health care includes understanding and honouring the body's natural processes and phases, and supporting an individual's innate capacity to heal. Our bodies manage trillions of chemical processes at an autonomic level at any one time. It keeps our heart beating without any conscious effort whatsoever. It has got it pretty well worked out in general – as nature does, unless it is interfered with. It knows what to do – if we could just get ourselves out of the way.

As the body, in its complexity, has trillions of biochemical processes going on at any one time, is giving a single substance – whether it be a pharmaceutical or a nutrient – to twig one or a few of these biochemical reactions, going to be enough to bring about a cure? To me, that is like throwing a snowball at Mt Everest! Good, natural, untampered food is what the body needs to support its physiological processes.

Nature is capable of generating a health-enhancing/survival response to almost any situation, and much of what we treat as a dysfunction is actually a compensation, an attempt of the mind-body to survive. The best that we can do is support these natural processes. Even the outcome of advanced surgery is dependent upon the patient's capacity to heal, which at some level includes their intent to heal.

We have become so detached from nature that 'earthing' has become its own form of therapy. Who would have thought that walking bare foot on the ground would be a form of therapy? When did we learn to trust new-to-nature chemicals over natural substances and give more credibility to something produced in a laboratory than to nature's abundant resources?

We have become so disconnected from our innate capacity to heal that we consider it entirely normal to only seek something *external* to ourselves in an attempt to cure our conditions. It has become a collective reflex reaction to look for that external agent to fix any symptoms or un-wellness. Thus, the burgeoning health-care industry!

Collectively and individually we have put much emphasis on what our bodies do and particularly on how they can malfunction. I do know that we have made big business out of it and have devoted a very large part of the economy, and our time an effort, to health - or should I say, *illness*. I often say that if I dropped onto Earth from another planet I would be amazed, and probably appalled, at the amount of focus, effort and proportion of the economy we devote to health care, how it so dominates much of our attention.

The 'great medical breakthrough' is not going to come from a laboratory, or from some unpronounceable new magic pill starting with X or Z; but from activating the healing power within us, and harnessing the power of our own minds. Thankfully we have evolved to a point where this seems possible, if not probable.

One might argue that the world in which we live is far from a natural, pristine state with the plethora of environmental toxins, polluted oceans, and contaminated foods we are all subject to. Might we just not be adding fuel to this unhealthy environmental milieu by getting further and further away from relying on our body's natural healing processes and upping the amp on technology?

It is a balance between using our health-care technology when needed, yet being as little reliant on it as we can, in favour of trusting and supporting our own healing capacities and applying very good self-care. When we get it right on the inside, we will be naturally more immune to and less affected by potentially adverse external factors. We will also resonate with and attract what is for our benefit.

We currently, generally, have a longer life expectancy than in previous times, and that is certainly in part due to our scientific advancements. But do you ever wonder how people live and thrive without any knowledge at all of biochemistry and physiology? How on earth did our species survive all those millennia when there was no knowledge of MTHFR gene mutations and such? How do animals survive without knowledge of the RDI of minerals and vitamins? Is nature just stupid and we have got to figure it out?

Modern health care is based on the un-voiced premise that nature and life can get it wrong and it is up to us to get it right – as though our limited human intellect, and our little tools of the trade, know better than the design of the universe. We health-care professionals (whether we are using sophisticated technology or waving crystals) can be so arrogant in our assumption that we know what to do. Yet, on the other hand, we are part of the design of the universe and we do our best; and better still if we align with that universal intelligence rather than our separate ego selves.

Why is it expected, and even considered normal, for people to be ferried from appointment to appointment to patch up various bits and be on a long list of medications when they reach a certain age? Does ill-health have to be a prerequisite for our timely passing from this Earth plane? Might we do better if we put our focus on what is working *well* rather than what can go wrong?

There is the potential for a happy balance between modern health-care technology and nature's way, between modes that relieve symptoms whilst also addressing the deeper causative factors. As we live in a time of abundant health-care choices this can, and is, being achieved by many. The 'best of both worlds' I call it, though I look forward to a time when both worlds are united. Meanwhile, we have to respect where we are, what we collectively believe at this juncture, and avail ourselves to what we have evolved.

So what is 'Mind-Body' Medicine?

The understanding of the mind-body connection has not yet filtered into our collective consciousness, and such discussion might sound like crazy talk to a lot of people. The practise of modern medicine is still based on the Newtonian model of reality, which views matter, including the body, in mechanistic terms. As previously mentioned, the belief in separation of mind and body, is still the dominant ideology in our culture and this is reflected in the practise of modern health care. And belief-systems do not like to be changed.

What really is mind-body medicine? It is a term that is thrown around and that has many interpretations. Some think it is the understanding that stress can cause illness and that methods to calm the stress will alleviate the illness. Methods to calm stress can indeed help, but they can also hinder by driving the root cause of the disorder further underground if a more in-depth understanding is not employed. Methods to calm stress, though appropriate at times, can be akin to putting a veneer over what is begging to be addressed.

Mind-body medicine is based on the premise that what we hold in mind, and in our broader consciousness, has a direct effect on the functioning of the body at a physical level. Thought affects matter. Constantly. No exceptions. We have been very conditioned to *not* believe this and generally consider the body as an entity separate from the more nebulous mind realm.

Mind-body medicine is not saying 'it's all in the mind'. Mind-body medicine acknowledges that symptoms and illnesses are very real and need to be appropriately investigated and treated on their own merits. The physicality of our bodies does need to be appropriately cared for and supported. However, mind-body medicine seeks meaning behind the illness, and is based on the understanding that mind and body are inextricably linked and that mind has dominance over the body. True healing involves looking at what we hold in mind/consciousness that is reflected in the functioning of our bodies.

Some think the world of biochemistry is separate from the world of consciousness. However, I believe the world of consciousness encompasses the world of biochemistry (and everything else for that matter). So giving a biochemical explanation for a disorder is *not* in conflict with the understanding that mind and body work together and that what we hold in consciousness influences the physical.

What goes on in our biochemistry and physiology is the *effect*, rather than the cause. There will always be physical manifestations and circumstances, for we live in a physical world. In the allopathic medical world we have just tended to over focus on these physical aspects of illness, often at the expense of the other levels of our being.

Most people still believe the causes of illnesses are environmental – what is external to ourselves, due to our genes or to random whims of fate. In fact, researchers from a reputable cancer centre in the USA have recently stated that two thirds of adult cancer is due to 'bad luck', with the other third due to hereditary and environmental factors. I did not realise 'bad luck' was a recognised scientific term! Maybe 'bad luck' means we really do not know. Think about it; how could nature get it so wrong?

A new understanding, through the study of epigenetics, has emerged at the leading edge of cell science. It is now well recognised that our environment, and more particularly our *interpretation* of our environment, has an influence on the expression of our genes. This has changed the concept of genetic determinacy. It is now clear our genes are not set in concrete and there are many influences on their expression. We now know our thoughts, which are part of our *internal* environment, affect the expression of our genes. We can no longer say the cause of an illness is 'just genetic', free from any impact from our internal mind/consciousness milieu.

It is largely unrecognised that the mind has enormous power over the body – positive and negative. The mind has a greater energy field than the body, and thus dominion over it. The body does not control itself. The mind controls the body. The body is under direct influence from the mind, via the brain and neurological system, as well as 'subtle' energy systems, most of which are working at a subconscious level. The subconscious mind largely controls the autonomic processes of the body. Every thought we have will have some influence on the body, positive or negative. How could it not?

With every thought there is a neuro-chemical cascade, initiated in the brain, which impacts the receptors on our cells and ultimately the expression of our genes, which then controls the structure and functioning of our bodies. At the subatomic level we understand that the *energy* of thought affects the energy of matter, including that of our biological systems.

From our experiences, conditioning, and conclusions about life, we might develop certain attitudes about life and related defences. These defences might shut down the natural flow of energy, our natural engagement with life and the balanced functioning of our physiological processes. In addition to affecting our mental health and wellbeing, these defences and attitudes about life can very specifically affect our bodies.

Our bodies are responding to our mind's interpretation of our prevailing circumstances, and this is related to what we have experienced and held onto from the past. For example, if the mind, and usually the subconscious aspect, feels that it needs more of a certain ability to survive life, this will directly affect the functioning of the corresponding part of the body. This is absolutely fine and necessary to a certain extent but becomes a problem if the concern, and need for compensation, is way out of proportion to the natural flow of life.

The physiological processes of our bodies continually attempt to bring the body back to balance, or homeostasis, for optimal functioning under prevailing conditions. Some of the compensatory mechanisms might produce symptoms, which can be labelled as 'illnesses' or 'diseases'. Then the 'disease' is validated and affirmed and is now seen as the culprit rather than being the physical manifestation of what is lying at a deeper level. The 'disease' is now the enemy to be eliminated.

Why do people have different diseases? Why is there such a variety of ways in which the body expresses illness rather than a general amorphous un-wellness? I pose the question: does healing just transcend illness because the new transformed personality cannot sustain the illness? Or, do we need to learn specific lessons from the specifics of a particular condition? Maybe it is both, or either, for different people at different times.

There are a number of people who have brilliantly and very specifically mapped out the mind-body connection in detail. They have precisely determined the link between certain thought-patterns and specific medical conditions. They have used empirical knowledge in addition to a clear understanding of anatomy and physiology and the human psyche. No doubt some have exceptional extra-sensory skills and tap into that broader field of knowledge that might transcend our normal intellectual understanding. They lead the way in this area and I pay homage to them.

The connections between mind and body are not always obvious on the surface and it takes a strong commitment on the part of the practitioner and client to delve into this area of health care. With all due respect, many people do not want to undertake this journey; but for those who do, it can be a very rich journey of self-discovery and health-enhancement. It is very important that clients be given the choice to proceed with their healing process according to what suits their needs and capabilities. Different healing methods and modalities might be more appropriate at different times and for different individuals.

It does take a bit of detective work to delve into the mind-body area of health care. We lock stuff into our subconscious for a reason, albeit sometimes a misaligned one; there is a natural resistance to opening up that 'can of worms'. However, bringing to conscious awareness our subconscious programming allows recognition that some of this programming does not serve us well regarding our health and our experience of life in general.

The healing journey is often about unravelling the misunderstandings and misconceptions we might have about life and ourselves. It is about gently loosening the defences, removing the masks and getting back to the essence of who we really are.

This is a process that cannot and should not be forced. One's 'being' knows when it is the right time to address the deeper causes of un-wellness. Many might never choose to do this. We are still developing the skills and language to tackle the mind-body area of health care and we are far from general acceptance of these notions. However, it seems a paradigm shift is happening and some would say long overdue.

Subconscious Agendas

The agenda of the body, and our primal imperative, is to keep us on the planet, to keep us safe – to *survive*. This applies as much, if not more, to survival of the family line or 'tribe' as to the individual. Keeping ourselves safe might mean very different things to different people and it applies as much to survival of our psyche or ego as to our physical survival. For some, keeping ourselves safe means avoiding any threatening physical harm; for others the emphasis might be more on avoiding rejection from family or community.

It all boils down to the same thing, and relates to our basic fear of annihilation; and with a different focus according to a particular person's predilections, experiences, influences and programming. For some people emotional rejection might be perceived as the greatest threat, whereas others might be more focussed on physical aspects such as illness or injury – whatever they feel is the greatest threat to their 'being'.

The subconscious mind is where we store everything we have lived through – every experience, every reaction to our experiences and all our beliefs and attitudes to life. It also stores our family/ ancestral influences and it is where we are tapped into the 'collective consciousness'. It is where we hold our suppressed and repressed emotional content. The subconscious mind, being much vaster than the conscious mind, is well and truly the prime mover when it comes to our health – and any other aspect of our lives.

The body will follow directives from the mind; and if the mind is largely below our conscious awareness, we are often *unaware* of this process. The subconscious mind, which is very aligned with our body's physiological functioning and autonomic processes, will sometimes go to extraordinary lengths for survival of the individual, as well as the family line.

The subconscious mind often has a very different agenda to the conscious mind and it has a tendency to hold firm to what it believes will maintain one's survival. Awareness of these subconscious/unconscious patterns can loosen their hold on us; otherwise it can be an exhausting tug-of-war, with two parts of ourselves working in opposition. It pays to know what we are harbouring in our subconscious mind that can so affect our health and wellbeing.

For example, if we are too busy, overwhelmed and losing touch with ourselves, and ignoring our real needs and wants, our mind-body in its wisdom might create an illness or injury to slow us down or push us in another direction. An illness or injury might be an acceptable way to withdraw from one's current life demands, if those demands are, in some way, perceived as a threat. If we just point the finger at the illness or injury we are missing the point.

We tend to think of injuries as just bad luck – wrong place, wrong time! And of course in our conventional reality they are. No one would knowingly invite an injury or illness. However, similar to any crisis, an injury can be a quick, if not dramatic, way of changing the direction in which one was going – physically or psychologically. An injury might also be the means of drawing our focus to an area of the body that is trying to get our attention, if that area represents some unhealed aspects of ourselves.

If, related to our current circumstances, we perceive our self-worth to be seriously on the line, and therefore fear rejection and significant social or economic consequences as a result, we might *unwittingly* create an illness so as to withdraw from the demands of life for a time. We are guarding our self-worth by not engaging in aspects of life that might make us vulnerable to judgement or criticism. If we do not understand this process, trying to force ourselves to heal the physical condition will be like whipping an exhausted horse. Is it any wonder that the fatigue syndromes tend to resist all attempts to heal?

One of the most common comments that any health-care practitioner will hear from their patients is: "I am tired all of the time." Of course there are a multitude of causes including environmental factors, toxins, over-work, inadequate nutrition, not enough sleep, and so on, and addressing these will help to a certain extent. However, we are all aware of the propensity for fatigue symptoms to persist in some people despite addressing these contributors. The *conscious* intent might be to feel better and have more energy, however the *unconscious body* imperative might be to slow down to conserve energy and withdraw from the ongoing stresses and demands of life for a time. Thus the fatigue.

Famine is one of the greatest threats to our survival and we are still biologically geared to cope with it even if we do not live in an environment where famine is a current problem. For some people *stress* equates to *famine* at a subconscious mind/body level. In response to this there will be a tendency to slow down the metabolic rate to conserve energy, and this might be experienced as fatigue and weight gain. This is the body's way of coping with the perceived stress and is very much influenced by constitutional types and genetic tendencies.

If we then go ahead, under those circumstances, and try to lose weight by employing rigorous diets and exercise programs, the subconscious mind might perceive this as *further* stress and then further slow down the body's metabolism in an attempt to conserve more energy. It will dig its heels in. Any conscious attempt to change might *subconsciously* be perceived as a further threat.

If we are lacking energy, as related to the above circumstances, and try to prop ourselves up with all sorts of nutrients and potions, this will only help to a certain extent unless the underlying mind-body determinants are dealt with. This is the conscious mind working against the subconscious mind/body and is very frustrating for the person as they feel that their body is failing them rather than trying to keep them safe.

When I see patients who are extremely frustrated, and even despairing, regarding their persisting ailments and concerns, and who have often been attempting to correct them for some time, I often sense there is a stubborn subconscious agenda working in opposition to their conscious desires. They often, and understandably, have a sense of desperation, and are looking for the one thing that will cure their condition. They do not necessarily appreciate it when I suggest their healing journey is a process with the mind having to be engaged.

This situation is often compounded by unresolved past traumas and disappointments and a pervasive, background expectation of more of the same. People subject to this dynamic might very much want good health but really do not expect that they will achieve it. Thus the desperation! This can indeed be a vicious cycle. Awareness will weaken the grip and allow some room for change of the fundamental patterns that can maintain un-wellness. We need to learn to work *with* ourselves rather than *against* ourselves, and ideally with compassion.

If one has subconscious guilt, this emotion, being of a lower vibration, can be a potent factor in the causation of illness. Subconsciously, guilt is calling for punishment or atonement. Along with guilt can be shame and apathy – all of very low vibration and life-energy depleting. These emotions are often the product of our response to our childhood experiences and our programming. They might be inherited and an individual's unconscious attempt to balance their family system. Subconscious/unconscious guilt will sabotage much of our happiness and health and it pays to address and relinquish it.

I do need to emphasise that this is *not* a conscious process but rather related to the signals that we are putting out from our subconscious/unconscious mind. We cannot blame our body as it is just trying to do its job in responding to the mind's dictates; however, we might look at the beliefs and attitudes we have been holding in mind, to which the body is responding. In this situation if we are just treating the illness manifestation we are treating the body's compensation for what the mind is struggling with.

Sabotages

In kinesiology we use the term 'sabotage', referring to the subconscious agendas that oppose our conscious desires. The question begging is: "What is the *pay-off* for not changing, or not healing?" We might want good health and success consciously, but what might we have to change, risk and give up in order to achieve these conscious desires? Please note, no-one is deliberately trying to sabotage themselves. This is an unconscious process that attempts to maintain our survival. However, we often maintain these patterns (which often start in childhood) beyond their usefulness and they eventually work against us.

When one has experienced an illness or condition for some time, and has adapted their lifestyle, social interactions and support network around having that illness, there can be a strong identification with the condition. This is usually unconscious and, at an ego level, there can paradoxically be a fear of annihilation if the illness is healed. Of course most people welcome the resolution of the condition; however, if there is a strong subconscious ego identification with the illness or state, this can be a hurdle that needs to be overcome for any healing to take place.

Jamie entered my consulting room for the first time and firmly announced that he had PTSD (Post Traumatic Stress Disorder). In fact he had had it since an accident experienced in his work place some twenty years prior. Though his physical injuries had largely healed, he had not worked since shortly after that accident and survived on compensation payments. Over the years he had many and varied therapies and no doubt gained much insight from those. However, none of these shifted his PTSD. He had a number of current health conditions that he wanted addressed. He gave the impression that he was very identified with his condition and would not want to relinquish it readily; and because of this there would be an unvoiced (and likely unconscious) limit on how far he would heal.

Probably he had not come across the right healing techniques that might have helped shift the trauma that was deeply held in his body/subconscious mind. However, a *determined intent* to heal, which will involve some change, has to be part of the equation. We are indeed creatures of habit and we can be very threatened by change of our state even if change is for our benefit.

The questions begging were: "Why have you maintained this condition when others, who might have experienced much more severe traumas, have fully recovered?" or, more so, "What are you prepared to give up in order to fully heal?" Often in these situations the injury triggered an earlier (and often long-forgotten) trauma that was not fully dealt with, resolved and integrated. It can be life's attempt to heal the original trauma, which is often blocked by our labelling the symptoms a 'condition' to which the ego might become attached.

Do we dare ask ourselves: "How will I now interact with the world and what will be expected of me if I am well?" "What responsibility might I now have to take on and what support structures might I have to let go of if I now heal my illness?" 'Wellness' can be a great threat to some people.

It is difficult to embrace full wellness when one is being compensated for being unwell. When one, unconsciously, attaches their very survival to the compensation received, and have long adapted their lifestyle around this, they can become like Rottweilers in holding onto the status quo. I have certainly learnt the hard way that people do not necessarily like having this pointed out to them!

As a health-care practitioner I am well aware of these subconscious agendas that can impede recovery from some complex, chronic illnesses and conditions. I have seen people get steadily better in response to certain therapies, and then reach a point where, for no apparent reason, it all goes backwards again. They default to their previous state. I am aware of the threat of 'wellness' to the system, though the client would consciously be in strong denial of this. In fact the medical system as a whole is in strong denial of this.

People can sacrifice their bodies and lifestyle to not face the truth of what needs to be addressed, though they might vehemently deny this. Illness is a great distraction from what one might not want to face within. Some people will just not go there and that is their choice. On the other hand, the experience of illness can also be the stimulus to propel one to enter and examine areas that might have been relegated to the deep recesses of their consciousness. This will give them a much more in-depth understanding of themselves and aid their return to wholeness and health.

These are very delicate areas to deal with, particularly as the un-well person wields so much emotional clout and is often put in this strange position of reverence. It can be challenging to address these issues directly with a person who is demonstrating un-wellness, especially as we do not as yet have a collective understanding of these areas. Again I do want to emphasise that the illnesses are very real. I am not suggesting that they are all in the mind; however, they *originate* in the mind.

It can be very confronting, and even politically incorrect to address these issues, yet this is where the real work on the healing journey is. This is addressing the 'shadow'. And it is not about rejecting those parts that are working in opposition to our conscious desires, but about accepting and integrating them so that they lose their potency. It is primarily about becoming aware of what can so affect us, and reminding ourselves of our fundamental innocence in the whole area of illness causation and manifestation.

Some might argue that mind-body medicine, the understanding that what we hold in consciousness can contribute to illness, is equivalent to *blaming* one for their illnesses. It is not about blame at all. Humans are innately innocent and because of this are very programmable. Very rarely is one deliberately trying to make themselves unwell. However, the subconscious mind will go to extraordinary lengths to preserve the psyche/ego, and sometimes at the expense of the body. The paradox is that we can unwittingly harm ourselves in our attempt to survive. There is no blame, but there is the opportunity for insight and understanding.

Often there has been significant past wounding or trauma of some sort when one experiences significant illnesses as an adult. The part of the being that is still impacted by the sometimes long-forgotten trauma is at a very different level to that of the adult intellect. The body and subconscious mind seem to operate at a level different to that of our adult, conscious mind. They speak different languages and often cannot reach the other directly.

Intellectual analysis of the problem is great for insight, but will go only so far and might not be able to get to the root of the problem. Methods that talk to the subconscious might have to be employed. These include deep meditation, hypnosis, kinesiology, acupuncture, homeopathy, chiropractic and many others. However, our *will* to heal, which starts in the frontal lobe of our brains, is a very necessary component. At some point it is a *choice* to heal and do what is necessary to bring this about. Paradoxically this can be the point of *surrender* to the healing grace of a higher order.

The intellect decides that it wants the healing to take place. If this is done from a calm place with strong determination and a willingness to do what needs to be done, then a healing path will unfold. If the conscious intent is clear and strong (but not frantic!), those subconscious hurdles can well be overcome, as the clear conscious intent will draw to it what is necessary to address the subconscious. And, it might come in various, and sometimes surprising ways. If the health issues are complex and entrenched usually a combination of healing modalities is required.

And remember, despite the experience of illness, most of the body is working well most of the time. Many of those autonomic body processes, which are so linked to the subconscious mind, are humming along just fine with maybe a few glitches here and there to sort out. At the end of the day, the over-riding force is to heal, to integrate, to return to wholeness; though there might be some very interesting twists and turns along the way. *Life* complies to do what is necessary to bring about healing – of the psyche, if not the body.

For some, illness is the mind-body's attempts to heal at a deeper level. For some, it will even mean death – not necessarily death of the body, though this can happen as the ultimate release; but death of the old self, the old way of being, and all that stood in the way of one's return to a connected wholeness.

Modern Health Care

People either believe there is a reality external to, and separate from, ourselves (Newtonian); or that 'reality' is a product of and a projection of our own minds (Holographic). These two different belief-systems give rise to two radically different ways of operating in the world and two radically different approaches to health care. Modern health care is still based on the Newtonian, mechanistic version of reality.

Our heavy and increasing reliance on technology has not necessarily produced a happier species as far as I can see. Stress is rampant and medical conditions such as diabetes and depression are endemic and on the increase. Morbidity and mortality related to iatrogenic causes is alarming and often ignored.

On the other hand, we have evolved some amazing health-care technologies that have prolonged the lives and greatly relieved the suffering of many, and it would be foolish to not take advantage of these when needed. Clearly there are some excellent scientific advancements, treatments and tools that can greatly help people with their health.

We are still in the chemical phase of health care, with its emphasis on biochemistry and pharmacology. Giving a chemical agent to affect a biochemical outcome is still (aside from surgery and mechanical treatments) considered the gold standard of modern medical care. It will be interesting to see where we evolve and further refine this approach; or maybe it has reached its zenith and will eventually become redundant.

Energy/mind-body medicine is still considered unscientific, despite much scientific evidence, as it is not based on the mechanistic, reductionist view of reality. The hard line, rational, logical, reductionist approach needs to be matched by an approach that encompasses intuition, symbology, and a 'bigger picture' overview. Both have their place and ideally work together.

There is the tendency in modern allopathic health care to segregate parts of the body and assign these parts to doctors who specialise in these areas. This has its usefulness as we cannot know it all and it is helpful to call on an expert, or 'specialist' in a given area. But does the body work that way? Does *life* work that way? 'The whole is greater than the sum of the parts', and *holistic* health care will focus on the whole, in keeping with a holographic, interconnected view of reality.

Surely it is our duty – and well overdue – to evolve beyond any out-dated approaches to health care. It has become a *habit,* and a very profit-producing one for some, to maintain a reductionist, segregated approach to health care. Simplistic approaches are sometimes very useful and appropriate but can often be an avoidance of the core issues. However, we need to be respectful that people are all living different realities, have different levels of understanding and have different needs and preferences regarding health care.

I have had many patients present to me stating they have decided to not continue with conventional medical treatments but would like a medical practitioner who could support their journey without judgement. Their health challenges have sometimes been cancer. These are people who have thought long and hard about their health-care options and have come to a conscientious decision, guided by what feels right for them. They are often considered foolhardy by the conventional medical world.

It takes great courage to go against the tide of popular opinion, especially when established institutions and authority groups back it. It also *is* foolhardy to not consider all options and avail oneself of the best and safest of what is available for one's healing journey. However, I consider that an intelligent, informed adult should be their *own* authority; open to advice from trained professionals, yet making the final choices regarding their care – if mentally able to do so.

As we are currently seeing with the vaccination debate in my area of the world, there can almost be a mob mentality at play when individuals decide against conventional advice. Though the groups that hold power are well informed in one sense, they are sometimes ignorant, or dismissive, of the full picture; and their reactions can be laced with emotionalism, fear and 'political correctness'. This is often hidden behind a rational and caring façade. Put simply, we can be conditioned and controlled like sheep and pity those who dare to stray from the flock.

There is just not a simple black and white answer to this debate and one can endlessly sort through the pros and cons. There can never be a hundred per cent guarantee either way, as life just does not work that way. There is no avoiding some risk, or potential benefit, despite the route chosen. But conscientious objection means *conscientious* objection. It is appropriate for authority groups to give guidelines, recommendations and advice according to the best of their knowledge and what they feel is best for the community, but it is alarming indeed when force or punitive measures are being applied to individuals who choose to not comply. Conscientious objection should not be treated as a *crime*.

Many people seeking non-conventional health-care methodologies have strived to uncover the causes of their illnesses from a broader perspective and have often trialled many and varied treatments and therapies. Some have done well and some have not, in terms of surviving their illness; and with conventional medicine alone, some have done well and some have not. There is more at play than the types of health care or healing modalities chosen.

I would never suggest that a patient not have conventional therapies for their illnesses. However, I do believe in individual choice and that an informed patient has the right to choose what treatments they feel are best for them. There are many compounding factors regarding these choices, as there are with illness outcomes, regardless of what treatments are chosen or not. It is just not as simple or as linear as one treatment brings about this result and another does not. It appears healing happens at a level that is more profound than just the negation of a certain illness or symptom and despite which healing method is chosen.

Of course we need as much evidence as we can reasonably get; but I again beg the question –"Who actually decides *what* healing is and what the criteria are for its objective measurement?" Is it removal of a symptom? Is it longevity? Is it a peaceful death? Is it inner peace or a shift in consciousness? Is it healing the ancestral line? Is it setting an example for another? We might never fully know and, despite some obvious commonly agreed-upon objectives, no single person or group should be the sole arbitrators of what healing is for another.

Should conventional power-holders punish individuals for their individual choices? In my opinion, no one group has the right to dictate what the populace should adopt regarding health-care practises. It is very important the client be given the choice to proceed with their healing process according to what suits their needs, wants and capabilities, if they have the appropriate information and intellectual understanding with which to do so.

Conventional medicine is very focused on what is wrong, on pathology. This approach is so engrained in our consciousness that we do not see it objectively and we assume it is completely appropriate. Of course we are looking for what is wrong so as to fix it – right? The reality is that if we look long enough we will find something that is 'wrong' and then label it an 'illness', which might then well start a cascade of expensive and invasive tests and treatment interventions. I have seen this again and again and have indeed been guilty of playing my part.

In a misguided attempt to be thorough and conscientious, and not miss anything 'wrong', we can very quickly put the patient in the 'illness' loop. Of course there is a balance between being appropriately thorough in our assessments and investigations, without being over-zealous – which is often fear based. Good health care also involves putting our focus on what is working well and doing what we can to further enhance that.

We have invested our collective belief into 'illness'; and (dare I ask) can we sometimes be a wee bit precious about our health? Overemphasis on the physical aspects of our being and fear of our mortality has contributed to our paranoia about health. We are often neurotically-obsessed with our bodies – in the sense of symptoms and what could be wrong with them, rather than viewing our bodies as precious vehicles from which to interact with life. It goes without saying we need to take good care of our health and ideally this is led by our intuitive knowing of what is beneficial for us, backed by appropriate knowledge. That takes some tuning in to ourselves at many levels.

Time we had more personal authority over our own bodies, health and lives. Being your own authority does not mean excluding appropriate health advice; but ultimately the health-care decisions should be yours, with a sharing of the responsibility.

Diagnoses

We tend to put enormous faith in diagnoses and labels. Of course they have their usefulness as they give us something tangible and defined to work with from a conventional medical point of view. However, we need to see them in their correct perspective and question the power we have given them. We perceive 'diagnoses' as though they are separate entities absolute in and of themselves. Diagnoses are labels applied by a person, or group of people, to observed, repeated patterns of symptoms and signs and their physiological correlates. This was for greater ease of dealing with the observed phenomena by reaching some consensus.

The labels then became sacrosanct and considered absolute. They developed a life of their own and were rarely questioned thereafter. We just believed in them. That is how the mind works. The unwitting expectation is that the person conforms to the applied diagnosis rather than the other way around. We have given too much power to the label and labels have a habit of drawing to them what is expected of them!

The predictions of how the diagnosis of an illness is expected to play out have become entrenched in our belief-systems and can ignore the multitude of other variables that a particular individual might be subject to regarding illness outcome. Our agreed-upon expectations, that are so habituated and fit nicely into our belief-systems, can help determine the outcome.

I was recently at a medical meeting attended by a number of international experts in a particular field of medicine. These were practitioners with a great deal of knowledge, experience and expertise in their field. They were considered top of their field.

Much of the meeting was about improving diagnostic skills in this area of medicine. The diagnostic criteria were based on recognised clinical visual features with supporting histopathology criteria.

In health care the consequences of missing certain 'diagnoses' are reprehensible. These experts, though obviously very good in their field, were not 100% in agreement with each other and not 100% accurate diagnostically (according to histopathology criteria). So who has the final say regarding what fulfils a diagnosis? If the world's top experts cannot be in absolute agreement, how can the rest of us?

What is overlooked is that diagnoses can never be absolute, though we treat them as though they are. The 'diagnosis' is not separate from the minds that create the diagnosis. A diagnosis is a description and there are many variables; and nature is not going to oblige by always presenting a condition in 100% reproducible form. Thus the experts in their field were not 100% in agreement. It is actually impossible that they are; as nature does not 100% reproduce what we have given a label to. We have projected a label onto commonly observed phenomena. Nature has not created these illnesses and conditions – *we* have, by what our minds have imposed upon these phenomena.

I have met a number of people who do not wish to work with a diagnosis as such because they are concerned that if a diagnosis is applied it would become a self-fulfilling prophesy. On the other hand, most people are relieved to have a diagnosis as it gives more definition and clarity regarding what they are experiencing, and they believe it can be more easily targeted therapeutically. From a practitioner's point of view, diagnoses certainly have their usefulness. We do need some definition and guidelines, though it helps to have some flexibility about these.

Rita came in to my office with some new and unusual symptoms that had some very concerning features. I had a very uncomfortable gut feeling something was seriously amiss; and so did she. Rita did not want her symptoms to be labelled as the suspected unmentionable condition, as she was concerned that psychologically this would work against her, as she knew the suspected condition had no cure and an expected steady downhill course. I later wondered if I had failed her as, following accepted protocols, I had referred her to the relevant specialist who confirmed the *diagnosis* we had both suspected but did not want to voice.

I wonder if the outcome would have been different had I not made that referral that put her through hoops of expensive tests, medications and procedures that did little to halt her eventual demise – as was expected from her diagnosis. The power of the belief in diagnoses, and illness in general, is beyond our individual minds and very much part of the collective consciousness that we are so very influenced by and can so very easily buy into; and it will take a shift at this level to bring about change in these concepts and beliefs. That might actually take some generations to come about and likely will be led by fresh, unconditioned minds.

We do not eliminate something by focusing on its existence in the first place. In fact we do the opposite. The sad reality is that when a diagnosis is made, one can live out the expectations of that determination. In the medical world we aim to get an early diagnosis so as to 'nip it in the bud'. Maybe if no diagnosis was made, no bud would have to be nipped. Consensus would suggest that this approach would be negligent. They would point to the many diagnoses that were made 'too late'. Well do we really know what the outcome would have been for these individuals if the diagnosis was made early?

Who Decides what is Normal?

"It is no measure of health to be adjusted to a profoundly sick society."
~ *Jiddu Krishnamurti (1895-1986, Indian writer, philosopher)*

Today, whilst I was at work, a very loud and garrulous patient attended the surgery. I could hear him clearly as he chatted to everyone in the waiting room. Manic I thought, definitely not 'normal'. When I finally got to see him I was amazed by his politeness, gratitude and general bonhomie. He definitely did not fit into 'normal' but he sure appeared to be happier than anyone else in the waiting room.

We can be so quick to judge and dismiss and decide that someone else's reality is not acceptable. People might be perfectly happy in their world that we have decided is 'abnormal'. So many people are medicated and counselled to be able to function again in a sometimes very dysfunctional society. I am sure a lot of them comply to gain some sort of acceptance and keep their place in the 'tribe'. Of course it is an entirely different matter if one's abnormal behaviour is a threat to themselves or others.

This also applies to psychiatric diagnoses – where a label is given to a collection of symptoms and where the original wounding might remain unaddressed. This is because it is uncomfortable for society to address its own shadow and it goes against our collective 'idealised self' to admit to such wounding. It is much easier to believe that genetics, the environment or 'bad luck' is the cause. We have collectively created illness by our avoidance of our deeper pain. Actually the avoidance and resistance *is* the pain; and the pain will dissolve when the resistance is lifted.

Placebo/Nocebo

Every therapy is a placebo to some degree. If, at a deep level, an individual really wants to heal, and has no obstructions to healing, just about any therapy will have an effect if there is the belief it will help. The therapy can be anything from surgery to an herb, and will be the catalyst for the individual's immune system to really do the job of healing. This can happen particularly when a 'treatment' helps shift the patient's focus from what is malfunctioning, to that of the healed state.

The placebo effect of many commonly used medications is now well known. The attitude and expectations of the treating practitioner is also a very important part of the equation. If the practitioner instils faith and trust in the therapies used and the patient's capacity to heal, this potentially enormously promotes healing.

During my stint in North India, I joined a medical team that was sent from Delek Hospital to tour the various Tibetan settlements in the state of Himachal Pradesh. This was related to the tuberculosis control programme that was run by the hospital. Our work included conducting health checks and providing education programmes to the communities. The hospital received various supplies donated from Australian hospitals and clinics and we took these with us when on tour. These would include a plethora of often out-of-date medications and vitamins.

I remember the faith many of the people in the settlements put into these 'treatments'. They were little more than placebos and a feeble attempt on our part to offer something to assuage their fear of their physical vulnerabilities and difficult living conditions. I clearly remember the sense of deceit I felt when dispensing orange vitamin C tablets as though they were the new wonder drug. Maybe I should have been more grateful for the temporary comfort they might have provided. I was certainly aware of the irony of using these tokens from the West in offering some form of therapy in an area of the world that has some profound and wonderful healing traditions.

It works both ways. If we are capable of responding to the 'placebo' effect, we might also be subject to the 'nocebo' effect, which is the experience of adverse symptoms in relation to an inert substance.

Jo was a young woman who came into my consulting room distressed by a host of physical and psychological symptoms that had plagued her for years. She was distraught, believing her multitude of symptoms were solely due to her having had a hormone-containing contraceptive device inserted some years prior.

Though the device had been long removed, she was adamant that all of her symptoms were related to having had it in place. She felt totally victimised and could not see that her beliefs and attitudes might be contributing to her problems; that her perpetual focus on her symptoms and blaming the device was helping to maintain the problem. In her mind the device was the cause of all her woes, and there her mind, for years, remained fixated.

This is neither to defend the device nor deny that some recipients can experience some significant adverse effects; however, clearly the power of the mind to exacerbate and hold onto the problem can contribute to the ongoing subjective experience of un-wellness. If we completely hand over our power to a device or chemical, or whatever is external to ourselves, we will also hand over our own power to heal the issue. When Jo realised her stress reaction to the whole situation was significantly contributing to her suffering, and she chose to put her focus on finding a solution rather than on the dysfunction, her condition improved.

What we project from our own minds onto a substance or therapy will significantly influence its effects – positive or negative. There is always a subjective factor; our minds are always involved, collectively and individually.

When we are so focussed on what can be given to us from the outside to heal our conditions, we will accordingly give that external agent so much power – and blame – when things do not go as we would have liked. Real healing is about igniting the healing power from within, rather than being dependent upon some external substance to do it all for us. This does not preclude the *assistance* of herbs, medications or whatever; but they cannot wholly do the job of healing.

Conclusion

We do live in a physical reality and our bodies might be the best way for us to learn what is going on in the other aspects of our being. As previously mentioned, your body might be the perfect vehicle for the feedback on what you are holding in mind/consciousness; your best means of learning on this Earth plane.

On the other hand, is there a reality, in life on Earth, where there is no such thing as ill-health? The acceptance of disease and physical vulnerability is so entrenched in our belief-systems and way of life that most people could not conceive of a reality beyond this. As so many systems and resources are tied up with the health-care industry some would not be too happy if these were not maintained. For many, their whole security would be rocked if those systems were not in place.

But why is it not considered a possibility that our bodies will just function well for most of our time span on Earth; maybe with some 'wear and tear' and ageing over the years, but not necessarily dysfunction beyond that? Most of us could not even imagine a life free of health concerns. If we can change or modify our beliefs and our beliefs influence our reality, why can't we collectively decide that illness is a thing of the past? I am just saying...

End of Chapter Points

- *"We are not so much meant to heal our illnesses as they are meant to heal us."*

- *We learn and grow through all of our experiences, including our health challenges.*

- *Our bodies can be reliable indicators of what we hold in mind/consciousness.*

- *Mind and body work together very specifically and what we hold in our mind/consciousness has very specific effects on our body.*

- *Much of what we treat as a dysfunction is actually a compensation, an attempt of the mind-body to survive.*

- *The experience of illness can help us re-evaluate our lives and bring our strengths to the fore.*

- *When we treat only the symptoms it is like taking the battery out of the alarm.*

- *'Healing' and 'transformation' are different concepts to 'fixing' and 'treating'.*

- *Conditions and diagnoses are man-made, not absolute in themselves.*

- *When we 'fight' an illness what are we fighting but a part of ourselves?*

- *Remember that despite the experience of illness, the mind-body is trying to keep us safe.*

- *The subconscious mind, being much vaster than the conscious mind, is well and truly in the driver's seat when it comes to health – and any other aspect of our lives.*

- *Subconscious agendas might be working in opposition to one's conscious attempts to heal an illness.*

- *People can sacrifice their bodies to not face the truth of what really needs to be addressed.*

- *Life and nature does not get it wrong – we just misinterpret it.*

- *Modern health care is based on the unvoiced premise that nature and life can get it wrong and it is up to us to get it right.*

- *When did we decide to trust new-to-nature chemicals over nature's natural healing resources?*

- *We carry our past, particularly the unresolved, unintegrated aspects of our experience, in our bodies.*

- *When one is very focussed on the physical aspects of their illness, they might well have suppressed the related emotional factors.*

- *We learn what we do want by experiencing what we don't want. Held within ill-health is the potential for sublime health.*

- *Time we had more personal authority over our own bodies, health and lives.*

Chapter 8 | # Love versus Fear in Health Care

"Love really is the power that heals."

ANONYMOUS

Some years ago I attended a talk by a well-known international author and spiritual teacher. He talked of 'love in action', of a robust, passionate, risky and dynamic love – a fierce and powerful love. He mentioned this was the love required to motivate positive change in the world at a time when it is so needed.

He was not talking about 'Hallmark' or 'Facebook' love or romantic or sentimental love. He was referring to that powerful driving force that keeps us 'on purpose' and in integrity to our truth.

There are many examples of individuals who have been propelled by, and who have exercised that powerful love; and who risked anything for its expression. Obvious examples are Joan of Arc, Abraham Lincoln, Martin Luther King Jr., Ghandi, and Nelson Mandela. No doubt, there were many others who have flown under the radar. They would, and did, risk all for a cause held much greater than their individual lives. We can harness that love to power our own individual missions, whatever they may be. And these missions do not have to be anything grandiose, but might be how we choose to be in the world, how we choose to treat this planet and its inhabitants.

I can scan a paper or watch the news on TV and read, hear of, or watch all sorts of tragedies; and sometimes I feel guilty for not feeling more anguish over others' sufferings. At other times

I can read, hear, or see a picture of something that touches me profoundly. That is the energy that propels me and shows me where to direct that love, and I have let go of that guilt by knowing what my cause is, and what it is *not*. And if it is not my cause, it will be somebody else's.

Interestingly, even though I work with people, it is the plight of animals that also very much touches me. It is something about their innocence. Some time ago I read of a story about the live exportation of animals. The story was actually about a sheep that, after its long and uncomfortable overseas journey, escaped the line-up when being herded off the ship at its destination. It fell or jumped into the water and was near exhaustion from swimming for who knows how long, when it was spotted by a boy, who led its rescue.

The people who saved the sheep successfully fought to keep it as the authorities had wanted it back. This sheep now lives a happy and free life on a farm, as a much-loved *pet*. To me this is an example of 'love in action'. Reading that story had me sign up for all sorts of animal rights organisations on the spot.

I also feel compassion for single parents as I have had some experience of this. I know what it is like to be exhausted by juggling the demands of needing to be both provider and home-maker/nurturer; of trying to uphold one's professional duties while coping with the ever-changing needs of growing children. I can relate to the experience of arriving home after a long day at work, having had maybe a 10 minute lunch-break, not to a warm meal put on the table, but to having to start the meal preparation from scratch, after a quick trip to the supermarket on the way home, and then assist with homework before tackling one's own studies and assignments.

I know what it is like to be entrenched in 'survival mode' with barely an ounce of energy to do anything but the bare necessities; yet be able, when the circumstances called, to get on and do what has to be done. As society is sorting out this dynamic, and hopefully evolving a better model, there are many of us – men and women alike – who are experiencing this lifestyle. My heart goes out to you and I tip my hat to you as you get on and do what has to be done.

I am particularly touched by simple human kindness; the real stuff that might go unnoticed, rather than elaborate demonstrations and Facebook hyperbole. The kindness extended when no-one is looking. This might be the choice to engage and smile rather than stare blankly; to say those warm, encouraging words rather than criticise or withhold. I often weep out of gratitude when I see images of the Dalai Lama as I am so moved by the kindness that he exudes.

We were also told, by that teacher, of some 'new age' delusions designed to keep us docile, passive and unaware of what is really happening in the world. A veneer of wishy-washy love to keep us dumb-downed and ignorant. The word 'love' can be so misinterpreted and misused. It can be used as a smoke-screen to cover what really needs to be addressed. It can be used as a righteous, 'politically correct' or syrupy mask to cover a cauldron of suppressed, unexamined content. He talked of having to do the 'shadow work' on ourselves as a necessary pre-requisite for dealing with the shadow of the world. I totally agree.

Many people claim to be aiming for 'love and light' but we sometimes have to wade through a dark, murky mess to get there. We cannot skip that part nor leave unexamined those areas we want to avoid. This is what the 'dark night of the soul' is about and is definitely not for the feint-hearted. We have this habit of projecting what we cannot own in ourselves onto others and onto the world in general. We cannot change what we do not acknowledge.

Fear is the illusion we have all agreed upon and built upon. Fear is a potent but misguided motivator. Fear is very controlling, as many politicians and religious authorities throughout the ages well know. We have been programmed to fear and I believe that it is time to say 'game up'. Our greatest fear is to be who we really are; free from the programming and conditioning that has removed us from our own authenticity.

As previously mentioned, our basic primal fears are: fear of annihilation; fear of change and fear of the unknown. These fears are different shades of the same thing and every other fear we experience is based on these. The job of the 'ego' is to survive, and it will do anything to preserve itself and submit to those fears.

Love and fear are the flip sides of the same coin. We need the strength of our love to face and manage our fear. The strength of the fear and vulnerability we face is also a testimony to the power of our love. The fear will sit on our shoulder as the *saboteur* ready to block our plans and creativity; but it will also remind us of the power of our love to overcome it. Love and fear are the light and the shade and sit in juxtaposition, both with a purpose.

Love really *is* the power that heals. All healing is the journey to self-love and self-acceptance, and acceptance of the role others have played in our development. It involves uncovering and bringing to light what we have harboured in our subconscious minds. This involves facing our shadow and integrating those rejected and lost parts of ourselves, and acknowledging the hurts and pains we have received and given. It means having the understanding that *life* is on our side, not our adversary; and that all we experience is ultimately for our growth and evolvement to a better way of being.

Forgiveness of self and others is very much a part of this process. It is also about changing what needs to be changed, standing up for ourselves and correcting injustices that need to be corrected. It is about recognising our own and others' innate innocence that is so easily distorted by our programming and so easily corrupted by fear. It is about being who we really are and being the *best version* of our authentic self – our own unique part of the tapestry. This is love in action.

This love is not a wishy-washy veneer of love but a strong, robust, courageous, inclusive and risky love. It is about taking off the masks that can cover that cauldron of unexamined content and looking the raw truth in the face. It involves acknowledging our programming and untangling the many influences that have kept us from the best of who we really are. It includes recognising the parts we have denied, rejected and projected and acknowledging our common humanity and the perfection in the imperfection.

Self-Love

All healing is the journey to self-love.

One's lack of love, or even hate, for him or herself is a large factor in the manifestation of illness. One can even carry a subconscious death-wish, which will sabotage every attempt to gain health and vitality. This can, in fact, be a slow suicide. There can be many subconscious factors at play regarding how we perceive and regard ourselves. We might well have internalised the messages we received, and the conclusions we drew from our early-life experiences. We might have then added a potent dose of guilt that caused us to subconsciously not allow the good, including good health, into our lives.

There might be a pervasive subconscious belief of not deserving, masked by a desperate sense of entitlement and a narcissistic approach to life. There might be the expectation that life is a struggle and if we are not in some way struggling we are cheating life and not gaining spiritual growth without enduring hardship. We might believe we will gain love and acceptance from others, and therefore keep our place on the planet, if we are self-sacrificing 'good' martyrs.

We might fear we will lose our friends and support structures if we demonstrate robust health and empowerment and change who we have been. We might value pity over self-actualisation and see it as a substitute for the love we did not receive in childhood. Our expectation of disappointment might overpower our desire for health and happiness. We might believe we are just not worthy of experiencing the good and just cannot have what others have.

Is this working for you? Do you want a better experience of life? These are all just beliefs, misperceptions, misunderstandings and the programming that is the *resistance* to our experiencing what we want to experience; and our misguided way of trying to keep ourselves 'safe'. These beliefs are not real, yet they rule us. Facing ourselves can indeed be confronting and can take considerable courage, but I do not know of another way. In my opinion, there is no way around but through.

The task is to observe, but not *identify* with, what is not working in, and for us. We identify what we want to change in ourselves – and thus our lives, without rejecting the essential whole of who we are. Identifying and dismantling what is not working in our lives needs to be matched with what we really do want to experience. We need to set our sights firmly on where and who we want to be, and what we want to experience, as this will entrain our efforts to this future state.

Paradoxically, a large part of this process is acceptance of who we are and where we are in the moment. That is kindness directed to ourselves. We are all a work in progress. It is not a race. It is not about some imposed version of perfection – another false mask, another way of beating ourselves up. I like to think that I am an *infinite* being; therefore I have all the time in the world to work on myself.

It is about matching patience with a quiet but steady determination. There will be ups and downs, as those aspects that are 'trying to keep us safe' will not want to relinquish their control readily.

We have invested a lot in who we have been and there will be some grief and confusion as we go into the unchartered waters of our new (or *real*) selves.

You need to work on this as it is in your cells. Nobody can do it for you, though they can guide and support. The real work is up to you. This is self-love in action. Bottom line – you deserve better. And what an exhilarating journey it can be! This sounds like serious business and it can be; however; it helps to also make light of it and not take yourself or your journey too seriously. As said, laughter is the best medicine; and we humans, with all of our foibles, are indeed funny!

Health is not just about caring for our bodies; it is also about feeding our spirits. Maybe more so. It is about healing the 'wounded spirit' and recovering passion for life – being *enlivened*. This is the most health-promoting factor of all. Better than any diets I could think of. It is very health-promoting, at every level, when you follow the path that gives you the most joy, and is most aligned with your purpose and your authentic self; meanwhile, knowing that *all* you experience is directing you to this path. Our bodies will be happy to co-operate when we do this; and will be the reliable vehicles, as intended, for our spirits to inhabit our humanness as we go about the business of life on this Earth plane.

Love your Cells

Our cells and our bodies respond to the right sort of attention, as we all do in general. Ideally we acknowledge our bodies and give them this *health promoting* focus. Not in a narcissistic or precious way, but in a healthy, caring and appropriate way. Everything in nature, including we humans, responds much better to the energy of love and gratitude than to that of fear and rejection. And primarily, we have to give it to ourselves.

Think of your cells and organs as having their own personalities and characters – because they do. Yes the whole is more than the sum of its parts, but the parts are important. Many of us go around as if we are (literally) in our heads with the rest of our body just trailing along. The brain is important and is mission control; however, I believe our mind inhabits every cell and component of the body, and our understanding and acknowledgment of this will help the mind-body to be a coherent, well-functioning whole.

The opposite of inclusion is rejection, and this applies to the body as much as to anything else. When we reject, rather than include and integrate, the outcome is disparate parts with disparate energies. This is not health promoting at any level; and we can observe the ill effects of this in society in general, as well as within our own bodies. Is it any wonder that a common cause of illness is groups of cells breaking away from their harmonious relationship with the rest and multiplying with no regard for the whole?

It helps to make a practise of consciously inhabiting our bodies. When we are *present* with ourselves, we will notice earlier when things might go awry. For example, if we are aware of the very first signs of a cold or flu, we are more likely to be able to do what is necessary to resolve it before it takes over. When we notice those first stirrings of emotion, we are better equipped to deal with the situation rather than becoming overwhelmed or going into suppression. 'Mindfulness' meditation techniques are very helpful in instilling the habit of being present with yourself.

Where the mind goes, the reality follows. If we fear and distrust our bodies, likely they will respond in kind. If we have the expectation they will function well, and we treat them well, more likely this will be the case. The 'law of attraction' states that we will attract more of what we focus on. It is an impartial universal law and does not distinguish between good/bad, pain/pleasure. If fear, drama, and painful tests, procedures and treatments dominate medical care, what are we attracting and what sort of picture of health are we creating with all of this?

Fear of our own Bodies

Having worked in women's health for many years, I have observed that the vast majority of women are uncomfortable with examining certain parts of their own bodies, such as their breasts. There is a fear of finding something like a 'lump'. This is an understandable fear, of course, given the prevalence of breast cancer and our focus on cancer in general; however it is still a programmed fear. In the context of health and illness we have been conditioned to fear these aspects of ourselves and treat our tissues like some disassociated and potentially disastrous parts. Is that health promoting?

Our bodies generally do very well at managing many complex processes. The resilience of our bodies and capacity to heal under some very testing situations is nothing short of miraculous. How often are we trained to appreciate, tune into, and care for our bodies in a loving rather than fear-based way? We can go to extremes to care for our bodies with all sorts of expensive diets, therapies and exercises; but if it is done out of fear, the body will respond in kind. If we are on a very restrictive diet out of fear, rather than being motivated by healthy self-nurturing and care, the body will respond to those fear signals.

If we choose what is nurturing and healthy for us, rather than focussing on what to *avoid*, the body will better respond. The same applies for exercise. There is a marked difference between compulsive exercise that is not really enjoyed and can actually be stressful, and exercising for the love of it. Going to the gym or going for a walk for the love of the body and the activity will hold you in much better stead.

I go to the gym regularly. Sure it is to get exercise and all of its inherent benefits; and to get out of my head and into my body. However, I go as much for the atmosphere as for the actual exercise. The environment reminds me of health and fitness – obvious, I know; but I feel healthy and fit just by being there, let alone going through the paces. I like the sound of the weights and machines humming in the background, and the happy chatter of people. I am sure other attendees feel the same. Some of the gym instructors are very skilled at elevating the energy as they coordinate the classes into coherent teams. Cheerful personality and elevated energy trumps technique.

'Where the mind goes, the reality follows.' I know if I am in an environment conducive to my feeling fit and healthy, more likely I will be fit and healthy. If the environment was stressful and antagonistic, more likely my energy would be depleted and I would not go back.

I hear a lot of health-care practitioners cite that 'sugar is poison'. We know that we over-consume sugar and that it is not healthy for us to do so, but do we have to put the fear of God into it? Trust me, if you do believe sugar is so malevolent then I suggest that you *don't eat* it, as you will be swallowing those beliefs with the offending food. Common sense is obviously beneficial but is extreme fear and avoidance really helpful? In my opinion, getting one's attitudes right is much more beneficial for one's health and wellbeing than any rigorous health regime. On the flip side, when we do adjust our attitudes to life, we will, by extension, tend to make healthy choices.

Are people healthy because they exercise, eat well and take their vitamins? Or, do they maintain these health-enhancing activities because they already have a sense of health and wellbeing and it is just a natural follow-on? Are people well because they eat well and avoid toxins? Or, do they eat well because they *are* well? Some might say if one's beliefs and attitudes are aligned with who they really are and with how life works they would thrive on a seemingly unhealthy diet; but if their attitudes are not aligned, and if there are significant ongoing or unresolved emotional issues, they would not thrive on the best nutrition.

Ideally we are interested in, and take care of our bodies in a non-fearful way. It is appropriate to be intrigued by what is happening in our bodies. How often do we sit in gratitude of them and the trillions of physiological and chemical processes that are keeping us on the planet? Fear is often programmed and really is optional.

'Primal' fear is normal and is obviously designed to maintain our survival. We are all subject to it; however, we need to exercise it in very few circumstances. It is common sense that prevents us from rushing into oncoming traffic, rather than fear. A reasonable level of vigilance and prudence is of course appropriate; and this, combined with self-love and the intent for good health, motivates us to care for our bodies in an appropriate way.

Healing Crises

Love will bring up anything unlike itself.

When we have been hurt and guard our heart from further hurt, we lock the pain in while trying to deflect more of the same. In our misguided attempts to avoid further pain, we also shut joy out. When the heart finally opens to love it will flush out the hurt that has stagnated there and one can mistake the old pain rising into consciousness as pain being caused by the current circumstances. It is the same with healing; the old pain will be flushed out, to rid our system of it and for it to be transmuted to a higher form.

Some healing practises describe 'healing crises', also called 'Herxheimer reactions'. We do not use these terms so much in the allopathic medical field but it would be very familiar to health-care practitioners of other disciplines. It means that when some form of healing takes place there will be an adjustment of the system, and this might temporarily produce uncomfortable symptoms; meaning, it can sometimes feel worse before it feels better. This is understandable, particularly from an energy point of view. It does not have to be dramatic.

Sometimes old suppressed memories and emotional traumas might be remembered, particularly if the client is in a safe, supportive environment. Sometimes physical symptoms, such as pains, might increase before they subside. It is well known that bodywork, such as massage, can awaken latent emotions and memories. Even the experience of surgery can open one (no pun intended!) to some profound mental, emotional and even spiritual experiences. It is a re-experiencing of what has been suppressed, denied or unrecognised for the sake of its eventual release and transmutation.

It is tempting to jump in and re-suppress these symptoms or add a new medication to 'treat' the 'new' condition. Sometimes a little time and support is all that is needed as these symptoms naturally resolve. Part of the adjustment is to change itself. It is letting go of the old and making way for the new. Like a snake shedding its skin, you might feel strange and vulnerable for a time. One can also experience emptiness when a profound healing takes place. It is not necessarily a matter of whooping around in joy, but sometimes a flatness or "what now?" feeling. We must be patient with ourselves as we settle into our new self and slowly discover the joys this new state will bring.

Fear versus Love in Modern Health Care

So much of modern health care is based on fear. We have been well and truly programmed to fear our bodies and the symptoms and ailments they might produce. We easily become suspicious rather than trusting of our bodies. In the context of illness we have been trained to reject and 'fight' those aspects of ourselves that are not optimally functioning. How can that be health-promoting?

Added to this are the fears inherent in the system, including the threat of litigation, the fear of 'missing something', regulation, control, bureaucracy, over-work, poor communication and lack of resources. This is a societal issue and is also reflected in other systems. The whole system is shrouded in control and fear – it is pervasive.

The practise of medicine is serious business. We are dealing with people's health, wellbeing, if not their very lives. Not much room for fun and frivolity in that! But maybe lightness brings more healing than a more sombre approach. The healing effects of laughter have been measured, and laughter might well fit into the category of 'evidence-based' therapies!

We tend to respond to illness with fear and urgency as though we are treating the enemy. We take the 'fighting' stance to combat illnesses such as cancer. Ideally, we take time to gain insight and understanding regarding the messages our bodies are trying to give us. It is best to lovingly work with our bodies and support them as best we can rather than treat them like machines that have been afflicted and thus in need of being 'fixed'.

All too often after one is diagnosed with a cancer, which might have taken years to manifest, one is on the operating table within days. This is often without adequate time to psychologically and physically prepare, reflect and really consider the treatment options. Treatments are often started in an atmosphere of drama and panic. We love the drama. Look at all of those medical television shows. We really feel like we are doing something useful if there is an atmosphere of urgency.

Particularly when in a state of shock and fear, one might very quickly relinquish their will to a higher authority. We can become like children when in this state and assume without question that the authority group knows better than we do regarding what is best for our own body. Fear and vulnerability will have one very quickly agreeing to some extreme measures. There is no doubt emergencies need to be treated as emergencies, but true emergencies are a very small proportion of the health issues that present for treatment.

On the other hand, modern health care has some amazing tools and technologies that can greatly assist people when they are facing health challenges. I have nothing but admiration and respect for my colleagues who dedicate much of their life to enhancing the health and wellbeing of others; and this is across many health-care disciplines including conventional medicine. I have seen how genuine love and care for their clients/patients can be so transformative and healing. When that attitude is brought into modern health care, with its utilisation of sophisticated technology and procedures, it makes for a dynamic, health-promoting system.

Death – the Unmentionable Subject

Modern health care is geared to keep our bodies going and alleviate the suffering that being unwell can entail. The downside is that it can be fuelled by our individual and collective fear of death. We have collectively decided that death is the ultimate tragedy to avoid at all costs. Our fear of death *creates* death and is propelled by our general misunderstanding and non-acceptance of our mortality.

Of course most of us want to have as long and healthy lives as we can and we will do what we can to achieve this – and so we should. However, our non-acceptance, misunderstanding and fear of death distort what we collectively do to care for our bodies. When we are not controlled by our fear of death, we much more embrace life. That is when we really live.

Some people spend so much time, money and effort on trying to avoid death they bypass the joys of life. Some people go to neurotic extremes to guard their health and will have every test under the sun in an attempt to ward off the inevitable. This is all to assuage their fear of their own mortality. It is actually a lack of trust in the process of life that fuels this fear and causes some people to take extreme measures to try to control the natural process of life. When addressing health (and most things for that matter), being run primarily by fear and avoidance never serves one well.

It is more beneficial to put the emphasis of health care on creating and sustaining a long, healthy, happy life, than on fear-fuelled avoidance of the unwanted. It is a seemingly subtle but important difference. We get more of what we focus on, regardless of whether that focus is conscious or unconscious. If we focus on health, we will draw to us more of what will enhance it.

It is very normal to have a reasonable, cautious fear of death, and a healthy attachment to living. There is a biological reality we are subject to and our biology is geared for survival. It is also very normal for us to do what we reasonably can to enjoy fulfilling, happy, and healthy lives. One's understanding of the whole life/death question will very much depend on one's philosophical and spiritual points of view, as well as cultural and social influences. This will be a little different for everyone, and we might agree that there is an existential reality, or mystery, that is beyond our everyday understanding of this subject.

'Jet'

We once had a cat called 'Jet'. Jet was a beautiful, purebred Siamese male cat that had exquisite blue eyes that would seem to pierce into your soul when they held your gaze. We kind of stole Jet. Well not officially, but I always felt we had. We first made Jet's acquaintance when he used to wander into our yard with increasing frequency. In his pre-'Jet' days he was a lean, wiry aggressive cat who appeared to be a stray with no fixed address. Very unusual for a purebred Siamese cat. Jet was enticed to our home because we had a constant supply of cat food; and cats did tend to adopt us. They would just turn up, unannounced, on our doorstep.

We already had a placid cat – a garden-variety moggie named 'Tazzo'. Tazzo was not inclined to fight Jet for his food. In fact, Tazzo had perfected the 'retreat is the better part of valour' approach to life, especially when dealing with neighbourhood cats. At any opportunity Jet would sneak into the house and go directly to Tazzo's food bowl and gobble down what he could in a few quick gulps.

Clearly Jet was hungry and was not having his basic needs of food and love met by his owners. We did try to locate Jet's owners, which included taking him to the vet to see if he was micro-chipped. He wasn't. We heard a long time later that his owners had gone overseas for an extended time and left Jet to the care of some friends – who clearly were not looking after him too well.

Jet became increasingly comfortable with us, as we did with him. He was becoming our cat, and we his people. This created a dilemma as we ourselves were about to move house and Jet was not yet officially ours. I remember deciding that if Jet arrived after we packed everything up and were actually ready to depart on the last day, we would take him with us. If he was not there – it was not meant to be. He was there – right on the 11th hour, just before we were to leave that house for the last time.

So Jet became our cat, and we his humans, as we set about to provide him with a 'forever home'. We officially adopted him through the local council after further checking there was no record of his original owners. By this stage Jet and Tazzo got along. They were buddies. Once Jet was provided with some consistent care and love he changed his personality – from that of a street-wise, fearful and sometimes aggressive cat, to a loving, relaxed, happy boy.

That experience made me very aware of the transformative power of love and care. All creatures respond to, and thrive better in the energy of love. Young children and animals, particularly, demonstrate this so well. Our cells are no different!

Conclusion

We are all going to experience fear at times, especially when faced with health challenges. Fear has many guises such as anger and aggression and many would understand that these expressions are really a cry for a deeper understanding, a cry for love. Love of self and others will soothe and entrain that fear. Compassion, a particular flavour of love, will warmly enfold the fear rather than forcibly suppress or discard it. Better to look the fear in the face and shake out those stress hormones as nature intended than hide them behind a steely façade.

When we are unwell it helps to love our bodies for doing the best job of which they are capable, at the same time as caring for and nurturing them in our attempts to regain wellness. True self-love involves accepting *all* of ourselves, including those aspects of which we would like to be rid. Love is working *with* ourselves in preference to resisting and rejecting those aspects we have judged as unacceptable.

Though fear might be a familiar companion for many of us, I believe that we are all incredibly courageous for having signed up for life on planet Earth.

End of Chapter Points

- *Our basic primal fears are: fear of annihilation, fear of change and fear of the unknown.*

- *The job of the ego is to survive, and it will do anything to preserve itself and submit to those fears.*

- *Love really is the power that heals, and all healing is the return to self-love.*

- *We have been programmed to fear our bodies and the symptoms they might produce.*

- *Everything in nature responds better to the energy of love than to that of fear and rejection.*

- *Our bodies will respond better to love and good self-care, than to fear-fuelled rigorous treatment programs.*

- *Love your cells!*

- *Health is not just about caring for our bodies; it is also about feeding our spirits.*

- *'Love will bring up anything unlike itself' – we call this a 'healing crisis'.*

- *Much of modern health care is geared by our collective fear and denial of death.*

- *The right **attitude** of care, combined with modern health-care technologies, can give rise to a very dynamic health-promoting system.*

- *When we accept our humanness and our mortality, we lessen our fear of death and more fully embrace life.*

Chapter 9

From a Physician's Perspective

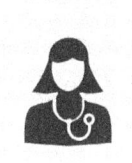

"No man is a good doctor who has never been sick himself."

CHINESE PROVERB

My perspective is mine alone and will be a little (or a lot!) different to that of anyone else. This applies to all of us as we all have our own individual versions of reality, even though there is much commonality and shared experience. My life experiences, conditioning and programming, family, ancestral and group influences all impact on who I am and how I view life – as does yours.

Regarding health care, I have had a particularly eclectic background and training, and this influences my views on the whole subject. I do not align with only one group. My bias is the mind-body connection and the role that *consciousness,* and thus *mind,* plays in our health as well as every aspect of our lives.

For me this has been a remarkably enriching and interesting, though often humbling, journey. I have very much enjoyed my studies in other health-care disciplines, in addition to the study and practise of allopathic medicine. I see no conflict in holding different paradigms of health care in my mind at the same time as they all have their place and are just different systems of belief and thought. Essentially, they all have the same aim – to heal. I believe that I have a fair idea of the pros and cons of the different systems.

One has a broader view when being able to stand back a little and look at different systems rather than being completely immersed in only one of them. It is difficult to see the collective beliefs, and habituated ways of doing things, of a given system when one is part of that system and has nothing to compare it to.

I allow myself the freedom to not be conditioned, nor defined, by any one system or field of thought. However, I do practise within the confines of a given health-care system, which is mainly Western medicine, as best I can. If I am representing that system I have to respect its rules and regulations to a certain extent. And when I am with a client, I am dealing with *their* reality and their preferences as well as my own.

I do not believe that any one health-care system has all of the answers, nor alone can deal with the huge spectrum of problems and dilemmas we humans can experience. I do not believe any one person, or system of belief, has all of the answers. We are in this together – this game called 'life'; trying to work it out as best we can so as to help ourselves and others through it.

Those of us who are in the healing professions do have extra training, experience and thus expertise in dealing with health and related problems; however, we are also in this game of life ourselves, subject to exactly the same issues as everyone else. We are not above the normal human condition.

Walk a Thousand Miles...

No one knows this job/vocation of being a medical doctor but we who work in this field on a daily basis. And, I say nobody can judge us until they too have gone through several years of high-pressured medical school, years of sleep-deprived hospital training, have established practises while raising families and generally trying to get on with life; and have been presented with thousands of patients whose myriad and sometimes very complicated problems have to be dealt with within very limited time slots. They cannot judge until they, too, have dealt with all manner of human problems and foibles, with nothing (including any body parts) 'off limits'.

I have sometimes been in a cafe and have overheard a conversation at the next table (not that I want to but some people are loud!) where individuals' medical ailments are discussed and where our profession is often scrutinised and criticised. I do not recall hearing similar criticism being pitched at the nice natural-therapies practitioners. Just this morning I overheard one such conversation whilst trying to read my paper; and all I can say is thank God that I was anonymous, and that I held my tongue! I am sure there is praise also but unfortunately some people are more inclined to criticise.

The conversations are often around what the doctor charges as their fee. I do not hear them complain about how much their hairdresser, plumber, dentist or lawyer charges. Not to mention what 'celebrities' might earn! This is based on the unconscious belief that those who work in health care have a moral obligation to serve, and that we are greedy or ripping off the poor public if we seek due compensation. I cannot tell you how many patients I have personally subsidised by reducing their fee and how many holidays my family and I have forgone because of this. Yes medicine might be a vocation, but it is also a 'job' and our means of income for the majority of us. And frankly, there are much easier and more profitable ways to earn a living.

We are often cast as the scapegoats for a general, collective misunderstanding of how life and health works. Both health-care provider *and* consumer are responsible for the health-care system as a whole. Our victimhood bias trains us to point the finger at what is deemed the authority group. Granted, sometimes this is warranted and necessary to bring about change. However, we are missing the point. Health care is a *societal* issue, not just confined to the health-care system but to society as a whole; and if there are problems with it, this reflects our commonly-held misunderstandings and misconceptions about how life works in general.

The illusion we have agreed on is, at least in part, driving the health-care system. Health is an aspect of life that is intertwined with every other aspect of life. We have mistakenly sectioned it off as though it exists unto its own, a neat separate category of life. It does not. It is because the whole area of health care is so tied up with our lack of trust in our own bodies, and with our fear of (and thus our trying to control) our own mortality, that it takes so much of our focus and is so driven by fear.

Who has the Last Word?

No one is forced to go to the doctor – it is not mandatory; though many believe it is. That is how much power the Western medical system still wields. It is generally accepted that the buck stops with the allopathic practitioner; that they are the final responsible group. 'All care, no responsibility' seems a little unfair to me. Let's just admit you do better at this and we do better at that and we can share our various skills and expertise and share the responsibility. For as long as practitioners of other health-care disciplines keep on assigning the final duty of care to Western-medicine practitioners (and for as long as we continue to accept), they will continue to hand the power back to allopathic medicine.

In my opinion, no one group or single practitioner should be solely responsible for another's health care. Even though this is how the prevailing system works, it is simply unrealistic. There might be a primary practitioner involved but ideally health care employs a team approach with *shared* responsibility. Different viewpoints and approaches are necessary for the overall health care of any individual.

I have often heard of people who have achieved a 'cure' by a particular system or practitioner, usually after doing the rounds of various health-care practitioners for years. The cure can either be from the 'alternative', or allopathic domain, and the conclusion is often that one system is better than the other. There is sometimes a triumphant sharing of the success and a shunning of the other profession. A broader view is that maybe *all* that the individual experienced on their healing journey was just what they needed for their eventual healing and the learning that helped to bring it about.

I am not trying to get into a slinging match, as it should be fairly clear by now that I have a foot in, and like to embrace, the best of both worlds. Actually, my aim is to integrate both worlds, as I believe they can truly complement each other, with neither party casting themselves as superior or inferior to the other. However, we also need to accept our differences, how we have each been trained and conditioned, how we are challenged in different ways and how we can complement and support each other. We are moving into an age of collaboration rather than competition. Let us make it a win-win scenario for all. The potential is enormous if we do.

Superhuman – Not!

I think it is fair that doctors are also treated like human beings and have the due consideration every human being deserves. That pedestal that we have either put ourselves on, or have been put on (and what a shaky pedestal it is!) creates the illusion that we are separate from ordinary human needs. This extends to assuming we do not having normal biological needs, let alone emotional ones.

I cannot count the number of times I have had a hurried 10-minute lunch break during a busy day; during which time I have had to make phone calls to patients and complete paper work. I understand this is not an unusual scenario, and is shared by a number of professions, and largely reflects how our society operates – though it remains inhumane. There can be a certain bravado attached to being 'busy', in demand and 'needed'; and we do get so addicted to those stress hormones! We consider this entirely normal and have trained our communities to expect this from us. We have created this situation ourselves and, thus, any change has to firstly come from within.

How did we get to this position of deciding we were beyond normal human needs and have our communities treat us accordingly?

The up side is that it does indeed build resilience; however, this can very easily turn into burnout, or worse, if the practitioner does not manage their energy very well. Of course there will be busy, frenetic times that we have to deal with, but this should by far be the exception rather than the rule.

It is very easy for the practitioner to get into the habit of not fully engaging patients when having to get through the day's long list. It is difficult to engage people at any intensity, one after another after another. 'Compassion-weariness' is a real phenomenon. It is very important to keep to those time and energy boundaries and it is so easy to over-extend ourselves (and trust me, I have learnt the hard way!) and run behind time, trying to play 'catch up' the whole day.

When we are fatigued, hungry and stretched and have that long list of patients yet to see in the afternoon, and hope to get to our son's basketball game in the evening – it is very easy to go on 'auto-pilot' and stick to habitual ways of doing things. There is a certain efficiency in being on autopilot, but not necessarily a lot of lateral thinking or creativity. We get by. We automatically put the blood pressure cuff on the arm, and know without thinking what to key in to order a test or write a script. We go through our oft-trodden paces.

I have had days where I reflect that I have been on 'autopilot' and 'unconscious' a lot of the time; but sometimes we have to do what we have to do to get through that long list. It is not the most satisfying way to practise however, and the risk is that some of those automated ways of doing things are not necessarily in the patient's best interests. Consultation time limitations have a huge impact on this. The recipient knows when genuine care is extended to them, rather than out of obligation or marred by exhaustion.

Though most people are very understanding and considerate, the occasional patient thinks that the practitioner has only one patient – them. They might have very unrealistic expectations of what can be covered within a single consultation and very demanding of a practitioner's time and energy. They can forget that they are one of many patients that the practitioner has to fully engage, advise, and treat within a day. Thank-fully these people are by far the exception rather than the rule.

The irony is that we tend to dote on our patients, while not extending the same level of compassion to our colleagues or ourselves. It is just not part of the medical culture to show any vulnerability, or debrief or muster support from colleagues. Though there might be some camaraderie, we tend to work as 'lone wolves', not daring to show our softer sides. We equate vulnerability to inadequacy. The boot camp of hospital-residency training instils that into us. We are expected to be above it all. For the sake of a professional façade, we will bury a lot of what is inherent in the human condition.

Contrary to popular opinion, our first responsibility is to ourselves (this applies *particularly* to health-care practitioners and carers!). We give better from a full cup. We should teach others the basics of good self-care by firstly applying it to ourselves. When we take good care of *ourselves* we are better able to care for and advise others – by example, as well as with the specifics of care. There is a more positive motivating energy behind what we do and more appropriate boundaries can be put in place.

Production-line Medicine

And who thought of having 10-minute consultations and running medical practices like production lines? Where did that come from? We can only ever deal with the surface stuff within that very limited time frame. It is impossible to properly engage, and know someone in any depth, within a few minutes. Is it any wonder that multiple tests are ordered and scripts written so readily? This is why practitioners default to micro-managing surface symptoms rather than getting to the core of the problem. As I tell my patients – whatever problem they present with has taken them a whole lifetime to arrive at. They bring *all* of themselves, including much of their past, into the consulting room.

People's myriad problems do not all fit into neat 10 or 20-minute bundles, though the system expects that they do. When consultation times are booked back-to-back there is absolutely no leeway for the consultation that inevitably goes over-time. We have all had the experience of the patient mentioning their niggling chest pain or bursting into a flood of tears as they are walking out of the consulting room! Thus the 10-minute lunch break – if we are lucky. People do not like waiting but a little understanding of the reality of medical practice goes a long way.

To review an individual's (sometimes very complicated) medical history, including family and psychological and social history, do an examination, sometimes procedures, order tests, issue referrals and plan management in 20 minutes or less is a herculean task to say the least. In fact it is impossible and only the most pressing issues can be addressed at any one time; and, of course, that has its place.

This leads to the fragmentation of the patient's care with repeated short appointments to just skim off the surface stuff and rarely deal with the person as a whole but rather a series of symptoms. Assigning different body systems and body parts to different 'specialists' further compounds this – as if our human system works that way. We can be swamped in a sea of test results, which have their usefulness, but this can further take our focus off the person as a whole. A person is more than their biochemistry!

Patients have also been trained to believe they can have their sometimes very complex health issues sorted out, and even cured, within this very limited time frame. They might come in with a 'list' of various symptoms and concerns, each of which needs due consideration and assessment by the practitioner. Sure, there are some simple things that can be quickly addressed, such as straightforward infections; but many patients' symptom-complexes take a lot of detective work to clarify and address.

I have had many patients present to me after doing the rounds of seeing various health-care practitioners to help sort out their often long-standing complex health problems. They are often very disappointed when the 'cure' is not offered in the first session, and do not necessarily appreciate the fact that addressing their health concerns is a *process* with a number of steps along the way. It can very much be like peeling layers off an onion. They have been conditioned to believe that there will be the one key to fix all their woes. It is no wonder that so many prescriptions are issued.

As I previously mentioned, we love labels and diagnoses as people like to attach a name and definition to what they are experiencing and the practitioner also finds some satisfaction in applying the label. However, this does not necessarily simplify the treatment plan. When we apply the label we then tend to focus on anything in agreement with the label. Confirmation of a diagnosis can be a long way from 'healing' the condition; in fact it can do the opposite when fixed negative outcomes are expected from the diagnosis.

It is often a disappointment to practitioner and client alike that medicine is more 'grey' than 'black and white'. Much of what a patient presents with, in terms of physical and psychological symptoms, simply does not fit the medical model, though many try to squeeze it into that format. As medical practitioners we are trained to quickly and definitely make a diagnosis and then plan all management around that, to confidently start the right treatment for the right condition. Obvious, right? I wish it were that simple! It would be if all of humanity's problems and experiences fitted into neat diagnostic slots (the DSM made a good attempt at trying!). It might be if underlying psychological and emotional factors did not compound human illnesses and conditions, and if all treatments were straightforward, without side-effects and quickly and completely did the job.

We know it is not usually like that and that iatrogenic causes of illness are significantly high. Much of the time, recovery from an illness or condition is due to the natural healing process, rather than, and sometimes despite, the given treatment. The treatment might be helpful in bringing to balance some biochemical processes and supporting the patient's innate healing process; and even buy time as the body gets on with the process of healing – or not.

It is a problem if we expect perfection from an imperfect system and *human* health-care practitioners. Of course, the 'bigger picture' viewpoint is the 'perfection in the imperfection', though this is not yet in our collective understanding. Every interaction, no matter how positive or fraught, whether it is in the health-care setting or not, is part of our learning in this Earth field. Every illness, regardless of whether it is cured or not, is opportunity for a deeper learning and evolvement.

Resilience

Resilience is a wonderful, life-enhancing quality that is often overlooked. It relates to our adaptability to life and circumstances, and our ability to forge on regardless. Our bodies are remarkably resilient, despite some significant challenges. Resilience is a quality that is very useful regarding issues of health. If you trust in your capacity to be resilient and adaptable, more likely your body will follow suit.

Medical practitioners are trained to be resilient. We have to be to deal with what we have to deal with on a daily basis. Why do we not also expect and encourage this in our patients? It seems that as soon as someone is labelled a 'patient' the rules are changed; this is based on the unvoiced premise that a patient is a victim of their own health issues and therefore should have special compensation. This can encourage pain behaviour which is wellness-defeating. The term 'client' changes the energy of the therapeutic interaction.

I recently did a general practice 'locum' in a small country town and noticed during my short stint there an epidemic of men dependent on 'pain killers' for alleged chronic back pain. Chronic pain is very difficult to prove or disprove. It is very often an entirely subjective experience. These men were dependent upon strong analgesics, including narcotics, and attended the medical centre regularly for their repeat prescriptions. Maybe their collective pain tolerance was very low; or it was an excuse for an easy means of relief from their daily concerns. All addiction (as with much chronic pain) is avoidance of the deeper issues – emotional pain. I was saddened by their loss of potential.

Why is it that some people recover relatively quickly from some very significant injuries and health problems, whereas others maintain the same (or less) injuries and debilities for decades? Could attitude, 'illness behaviour' and avoidance of the deeper issues be playing a role? I am not saying there are not some potent health challenges the majority of people would struggle with; however, some people will muster their determination and resilience to deal with them, while others will very quickly go into defeatism and look for the easy way out.

Health care in general is geared to relieving pain and suffering; but might we be inadvertently prolonging it, by driving further underground the real issues and causation, in our attempts at symptom control? There is a great deal of political correctness about relieving pain and symptoms, and sometimes self-righteous expectation of such from the health-care consumer. This is entrenched in our medical system and the pressure of the health-care practitioner to abide by this is very compelling indeed. Meanwhile, the commonly associated emotional traumas go unaddressed.

Of course we want to relieve people's suffering and have them return to a sense of health and wellbeing; but, as those men in that small town demonstrated, just addressing the surface symptoms is a long way from achieving that.

We are so wary of suggesting that attitude is a significant, and often overlooked, causative factor in illness, or at least in the *experience* of illness. Attitude is based on personal and collective beliefs, which in turn are related to unintegrated and unresolved life experiences and related misunderstandings about life. Do we dare go there? Difficult to do in a 10-minute consultation!

Some people are very willing to be accountable and address all of themselves; some others firmly close the door on that and put their energy and focus on the diagnosis. Illness can be a great distractor from other aspects of our being; and much easier to point the finger of blame rather than do the real work and be accountable for ourselves and our role in the healing journey.

Sometimes people have to be confronted if all else fails. Personally, the times when I have most taken note and made some necessary changes in my life (or more so my attitudes), is when I have been confronted. Very uncomfortable at the time, and tempting to go into victim mode and lick my wounds, but often the jolt that I needed to wake up and have a good look at myself. I applaud the courage of the people who have directed me to look at the truths that I had so wanted to avoid.

This needs to be done with compassion and skill, with the client's best interests always in sight. There does need to be flexibility around this and we need to do, in the moment, what feels right for both patient and ourselves. It is quite a balancing act. However, the more we 'rescue', the more we are promoting the victimhood and helplessness of the patient. This arrangement suits some people quite well, but at the risk of forgoing empowerment of both parties.

Some of you might be aware of the 'butterfly story'. It goes something like this… A man was walking with his young son in a forest when they came across a butterfly trying to release itself from its cocoon. The boy asked the father to help free the butterfly by opening the cocoon with his penknife. The father acquiesced and the butterfly fell out of the cocoon with small, undeveloped wings and a swollen body. It was clear it would not be able to fly, and thus not survive.

The father explained to his son that they had jumped in and helped too soon, as the butterfly needed to struggle through the tight cocoon to remove the fluid from its body and have its wings more fully develop. It is similar with the human condition – sometimes we, health-care professional or not, jump in too soon to 'rescue', and because of this do not allow the other to learn what they might have if we had stood back a little.

Healer, Heal Thyself

The ideal health-care practitioner is the one who is whole and integrated in him or herself, with no significant unresolved issues that might unconsciously play out in the practitioner-patient relationship. Realistically there are probably very few people who can boast that. There is no doubt that many who are attracted to the healing arts, have themselves something to heal. As is said, 'healer heal thyself' and 'we teach what we most need to learn'.

If this is unconscious it can be harmful, if not dangerous, for all involved. If the practitioner has consciously been through their own healing journey they are more likely to be aware of the pitfalls and challenges involved and know what is achievable. The bigger picture is that we are all trying to heal or integrate something. We are all learning and upgrading our understandings at all times. That is life on planet Earth.

I do not know if it is possible to take someone on a healing journey from a lofty position of being separated and above it all. Of course non-attachment and objectivity is necessary to a large degree, but not at the expense of hiding behind a mask of superiority. At the end of the day we are all humans sharing this human experience and I do not think many people have reached a completely healed state; or, indeed, if such a state even exists.

The best we can do for our patients comes from our being the very best and most healed version of ourselves that we can be. This, paradoxically, includes accepting the flaws and foibles that are inherent in our human condition. Aiming for that healed state can be a life journey for many of us, rather than something that can be achieved in a weekend course.

Sometimes we trade our humanness for that mask of professionalism. For those of us who are 'perfectionists' (and that is a large percentage of those who are in the medical profession) it feels very threatening to admit to any vulnerability. It is so 'unprofessional'. Even to admit that we do not know something can bring on panic attacks!

I was at a medical meeting some time ago where a number of doctors expressed the importance of never showing their vulnerability in the work setting. That seems very reasonable and expected behaviour; yet, appearance and image seemed to be more important than truth. Why do you think many doctors shut down on their own emotions and their hearts and work in an automated way? I am not saying we go around having histrionic fits and spilling everything out, but that we are at least aware and accepting of our own humanness – which includes some normal vulnerability at times.

Professionalism is a worthy ideal, and one we should attempt to uphold; but it can be yet another mask that we hide behind to conceal our shared humanness – and mainly from ourselves. One *does* have to maintain a certain objective overview of other people's problems and reality; and there is indeed a fine line between empathy and sympathy. Of course the focus is on healing and empowering the patient, while drawing on our own knowledge and life experience to that end.

Empathy comes from sharing the human experience, from having some understanding of what others might be experiencing and how to best navigate through it. One of the most beneficial things that a health-care practitioner can do for the client is to be fully *present* with them, to give them their undivided focus, with their very best interests at heart. It is difficult to do this if we have little understanding of what they are experiencing.

In life we help and influence others most by our example; and this can be the example of what *not* to do as much as what to do. Like any humans, health-care practitioners of course have their own challenges and issues to deal with. No doubt this can promote empathy for others' plights; however, the task is to find a way through these and then teach by example. That is often the healer's journey.

The health-care practitioner's unresolved issues should not influence interactions with their patients; so it is the duty of any health-care professional to sort him or herself out as best they can, and with the aid of other professionals if needed. However, we have to have a degree of self-awareness to recognise if any issues are there to be addressed in the first place. The more self-aware the professional is, the less they will project their own issues and biases into the consultation. It can be very humbling indeed for those of us who are meant to be above it all, to admit to, and seek help for our own physical and emotional vulnerabilities.

Health-care practitioners can project their fear of their own mortality onto their clients, and onto the health-care system as a whole. Sometimes overzealous and maybe extreme or even inappropriate treatments can reflect the unacceptance of our human mortality, and the belief that death is always wrong and avoidable. Personally I believe that quality of life trumps duration of life; though obviously we aim for both.

Taking on the role of health-care professional, or 'healer', is actually a very unnatural process, as it inevitably puts us apart from our fellow human beings – whilst we are not apart from our common humanity. It can be a heavy, heavy burden to feel solely responsible for another's health and wellbeing, especially when this does not resonate with the truth of *self-responsibility*. It is convenient for society to have a group to which they can hand over their personal responsibility and afford blame to when the outcome is not as they would have liked. Is it any wonder that the rate of suicide, depression and alcohol abuse is disproportionally high in our profession?

Self-Care for the Practitioner

There is an unspoken tendency in our profession to be seen as being able to do the 'hard yards'. Particularly during those early hospital-training years there was absolutely no point in complaining about long hours and sleep deprivation. Clearly the culture was to tough it out and tuck it all under our belts; an 'initiation' into the world of medicine, so to speak. Our superiors supposedly did it even tougher (though, I do not know how!) and it was to our detriment regarding future employment to appear wussy or complain. No fluffy de-briefing and group hugs back when I went through my hospital-training years!

I remember that during my intern days I was very judgmental of a colleague who actually took time off work because of illness. What an indulgence! I remember working those horrendous, stressful hours with the flu and all manner of illnesses, believing I could not demonstrate any weakness. That *was* my weakness. How many times have doctors sat in their consulting room feeling very unwell, dispensing sick leave certificates to patients who seemed to be fairing a lot better; and helping patients with work-related 'stress leave' when they would never consider going down that path themselves?

I choose to limit the days I practise medicine. I am of no value to anyone if I am burnt-out and practise a sub-standard, reflex-type medicine because I am too exhausted to think laterally. I also have many other interests I like to pursue to create a balanced life. I do know there are many health-care practitioners who are extremely dedicated to their craft, pretty much put it above everything else in their lives, and are almost continuously 'on call'. I greatly admire their tenacity and dedication.

I give 100% to my patients when I am available, and spend countless extra-curricular hours studying and attending workshops and seminars – as we do. However, my own time is my own time; I need a balance in my life, and there are other ways I like to spend my time. There is an unwritten and unvoiced code that we are only worthwhile practitioners if we martyr ourselves to the profession and make everything else secondary. Medicine is a 'vocation' after all. If that is what is required, then I guess I do not have what it takes.

There is also a modern-day tendency to keep up with the research. This alone could be a full-time job, given the plethora of information available. Some professionals are simply fascinated by research and want to continually upgrade their knowledge for the benefit of their patients and for their own intellectual interest. But, who goes fishing anymore? Where did simplicity go? Is life meant to be this frenetic; and have we proven that pouring over the latest research findings for hours and attending countless seminars actually *improves* the quality of life for our patients or ourselves?

'I prefer to Know that you Care than Care what you Know.'

Part of any healing is 'holding the space' and validating another's experience in this game called 'life'. It is about sharing the commonality of the human experience and holding the highest vision for the client. When you present to a health-care/healing practitioner, you are going to present with your problems and wounded-ness for this is what you want to address and overcome. This is indeed a vulnerable state especially if the person you are entrusting with your care, your body, and sometimes our innermost secrets, is a virtual stranger.

I believe it is one of the greatest privileges to 'bear witness' to another's experience, to be entrusted to hear their life story and their concerns, and to then care appropriately. Health-care professionals are in the position of allowing others to share with them what they might not have been able to express to anyone else on this earth, and then help as best they can. The one seeking assistance needs to discern which practitioner they can entrust their health concerns with.

I once heard a very wise individual say that the best thing we can do for our patients is to see them as whole, complete and perfect as they are – *inclusive* of their illnesses. Though this can indeed be a challenge when the patient is very unwell and has complex health problems, the practitioner needs to know there is another side to their patient. It is helpful to have the potential healed and whole state of them in view.

We cannot heal if we only focus on pathology. We have to envision the healed, whole state of the individual as best we can while, paradoxically, seeing the perfection in their current condition. This is not necessarily easy, as we have been so trained to take a different perspective.

It is said that various spiritual masters saw only the healed state in the one wanting to be healed; this then did not allow any room for the illness. We are so focussed on fixing and healing that we rarely see the perfection in their current state. It is something I aspire to but have a long way to go yet.

Intuition in Health Care

In the consulting setting, health-care professionals are receiving intuitive information about their clients all of the time, though some would not necessarily call it that. Whether we listen to it is another matter. Because health-care practitioners work so closely with people and get into the habit of tuning into them, they hone their intuition over the years. Many decisions will be made in a gestalt fashion, which includes that 'inner knowing' in addition to our knowledge-base. This happens quickly and subliminally. Our intuition is inclusive of, but more expansive than, our knowledge-base and experiential information.

The practise of medicine, as with all health-care professions, is also an art; and intuition plays a very big part in how physicians choose to treat their patients. In the pre-technology days, physicians would almost exclusively rely on experience and intuition – and became very skilled at it. The more tools we have and tests we do, the less reliant we feel we need to be on our deeper, and even common sense, knowing. It is so easy to focus on a plethora of sophisticated test results whilst losing sight of the 'is-ness' of the person sitting in front of us.

I often have patients present to me with folders of extensive test results and who can discuss the intricacies of their biochemistry and cite the latest research in detail. This has its place, but it saddens me that they might not be so well-versed regarding their inner emotional world, their values and purpose, and the meaning they put on their own lives. It alarms me when we treat ourselves, or others, as machines needing to be fixed.

We have risked removing ourselves from what used to be an integral part of any therapeutic relationship by bowing down to technology and deciding the world of science is superior to the more intangible aspects of human interaction. The best of modern medicine is a combination of both healing art and science.

Despite obvious commonality, no two people are alike, and nor will be the therapies to which they best respond. We love procedures and protocols and stock-standard ways of doing things. They clearly have their usefulness and are good as guidelines; however, it is not always a matter of 'one size fits all'. It is a sad thing when fixed protocols get in the way of what one intuitively knows is best for one's clients.

My training in kinesiology exposed me to a very different approach to health care. Kinesiology employs muscle testing as a bio-feedback tool to access the client's whole system including their subconscious mind. The biofeedback will guide the practitioner to the 'where, what and why' underlying the client's issue, and to what remedies might be of benefit for them. It is a very individual process and is based on the understanding that we are all unique and might require different approaches and remedies at different times.

As a health-care practitioner, if I was really courageous and had my patient's very best interests at heart, I would work with that person intuitively. I would say what I felt needed to be heard and initiate treatments I felt were best for that person in the moment. I would be *guided* by 'evidence-based' practises and protocols, however they, or any statistical analyses, would not control how I practise. After all, I am dealing with the individuality of the person in front of me.

What I felt was best for that person would not be controlled by fear of litigation and straying from the status quo; though I would adhere to recommended practises as best I can. I believe that is what integrity is – doing what one truly believes is right in the moment despite views from the majority that might disagree. This I aspire to but I am not quite there yet. There is still a certain amount of looking over my shoulder.

Conclusion

As previously mentioned, I believe that 'life' is the greatest teacher, and that the main role of the therapist is to assist the client in understanding this. The doctor, therapist, health-care practitioner can use their training and expertise to facilitate and guide another's care; however do we *really* know what is in the client's best interests? Do we believe that we know better than the design of the universe? We do our best, given what we know, and according to our craft and the system we work within; but ideally with some humility and understanding that we really are just bit-players in a much larger field.

What we put our focus on we get more of – until we decide to adjust our focus. The health-care industry collectively has made a very good and convincing job of putting our focus on pathology – what is *wrong* with our bodies and ourselves. By extension, individuals then tend to put their focus on what is wrong, or can go wrong, with their own bodies, rather than on abundant good health. If we swung the pendulum to focus on what is *right* about ourselves, including our experience of illness, its inherent learning *and* our potential to be healthy no matter what, we might have a very different collective outcome.

Better to teach people to be health-focussed, rather than illness-focussed, to see their own potential to be well. This might seem a bit Utopian, but we know that we humans are capable of monumental changes when we decide to take that initiative.

The practise of medicine is serious business. Hospitals and doctor's surgeries are not the happiest of places, and that is understandable as people are often dealing with some significant health concerns. Is it irreverent and disrespectful to wish that some fun might sneak in somewhere? Dare I wish to have some lightness and joy in the process? Well suffering begets suffering and fear begets fear, just as lightness and joy begets lightness and joy. Let's aim for a happy balance of seriousness, focus and some lightness to boot.

In my opinion, education is the key. How people look after themselves generally, as well as their expectations of the healthcare system, need to be addressed. This is more of a global issue. It is very easy to scapegoat one group; yet they are but part of the whole interactive societal system. Fundamentally, it is our beliefs about the whole subject of 'health', and life in general, that underlies how this system operates. It is our understanding of how life works, including the *meaning* we assign to our experiences and health challenges, that is at the core of the problem – and of the solution.

End of Chapter Points

- *No one health-care system has all of the answers.*

- *We are all in this game of life together trying to help each other as best we can.*

- *No-one, including the health-care practitioner, is above the human condition.*

- *Health care is a societal issue, not just confined to the health-care system but to society as a whole.*

- *The health-care system and its practitioners can be cast as the scapegoats for a general, collective misunderstanding of how life and 'health' works.*

- *It is because the whole area of health is so tied up with our lack of trust in our own bodies, and with fear of our own mortality, that it takes so much of our focus.*

- *For the sake of a professional façade, health-care practitioners will bury a lot of what is inherent in the human condition.*

- *Resilience is a quality that is very useful regarding issues of health; and is to the benefit of both health-care practitioner and client.*

- *It is often a disappointment to practitioner and client alike that medicine is more 'grey' than 'black and white'.*

- *Regarding health care, it is not always a matter of 'one size fits all'.*

- *The more tools we have, the less reliant we feel we need to be on our deeper, and even common sense, knowing.*

- *The best thing we can do for our patients is to see them as whole, complete and perfect as they are.*

- *Better to teach people to be health, rather than illness-focussed, to see their potential to be well.*

Epilogue | **White Christmas**

Many years ago, in fact in 1985, I experienced my one and only white Christmas. Now this was neither in North America nor Europe. It was in India, in the foothills of the Western Himalaya, near the small village of McLeod Gang, in the state of Himachal Pradesh.

As a young doctor I had travelled to India to do volunteer work at a small hospital in Dharamsala, the capital of Tibetans in exile. I had travelled to India the year before and fell in love with this amazing country and dreamed of returning to work there. Several months after my return to Australia, a colleague rang me out of the blue asking if I would be interested in working in North India. This would involve work at a small hospital –Delek Hospital, which had had a long tradition of Australian volunteer doctors. I went, without a moment's hesitation nor a backwards glance.

It was difficult to explain what appeared to be a very irrational move away from a secure job, into the unknown, on a whim. I have certainly had my impulsive moments; and maybe this was one of them. But it felt much deeper than that. This felt like a calling, beyond and regardless of logic. I went, like a moth to the light. India had called and I had responded.

The journey was long and uncomfortable on many levels. This was in the day of hand-written letters. All I knew was that I was going to a small hospital in a place called Dharamsala, in North India. There was no website to check nor emails to detail and confirm my position. There was no volunteer organisation involved to support me and watch my back, no companion with whom to share the journey. I was going it alone on the back of a whim. I was ready for adventure and India had beckoned.

I had grasped this opportunity to broaden my medical experience and, more so, to learn about life. I had no illusions that my contributions would not be far out-weighed by the learning gained. The experience made me question many of the dogmas to which I had previously been conditioned, and it indeed changed my worldview. Previous to this experience I had been cynically dismissive of anything other than my conventional Newtonian version of reality. I knew in my heart that I was drawn to this place to question what was previously unquestionable.

Dharamsala was very difficult to get to in those days and, for all I know, it might still be. After arriving in Delhi there was a long, overnight bus ride along some quite treacherous roads to Dharamsala, much further up north. I remember sitting alone on that rickety bus, as it rocked to 'Bollywood' movies for the whole journey, alone, the only foreigner on the bus, in the middle of who knows where, stomach churning from who knows what I ate, travelling to who knows what experiences, looking out into the darkness pondering – 'What *was* I thinking?'

On my arrival I was greeted by the hospital driver in his trusty jeep. I would get to know that jeep very well as it was the hospital's only means of transport and doubled as ambulance and patient and staff transit. It would drive me through a smorgasbord of adventures. Sleep deprived, with guts in a delicate state and still overwhelmed by India's cacophony of colour, sound and movement, I had arrived.

This place and its people instantly felt familiar to me and I very soon felt at home. At the same time, all seemed so exotic and new. I worked and lived at Delek Hospital, a small hospital run by, and for, Tibetan refugees. My small, blue-painted room was above the tuberculosis ward. I ate the same food as the patients, mostly rice and dhal, and bathed for six months out of a bucket of heated water. Going into town for Tibetan mo-mos and Indian sweets was a treat. I spent a lot of time with the hospital staff and their families and this gave me some understanding of these wonderful people and their cultures. I also developed a strong camaraderie with my fellow volunteer doctors.

As well as being the capital of Tibetans-in-exile, this area was the heart of Mahayana Buddhism in India. In addition to the Dalai Lama's monastery, many smaller monasteries dotted the area. On our regular trips to McLeod Gang further up the foothills, we would see gaggles of monks and nuns, in their distinctive maroon and gold robes, walking to and from their monasteries. In addition to the local Indian and Tibetan populace, this area was also home to a spattering of Western spiritual seekers, adventurers and hippies. The exciting blend of cultures gave great colour to this pocket of Himachal Pradesh.

I had befriended some 'Dharma Junkies', as Western Buddhist spiritual seekers were sometimes affectionately known in those areas. Some of them, being advanced students, were fluent in the Tibetan language. My new friends helped me explore the local terrain and helped open my eyes to another world and another way of being.

I would sometimes accompany them to visit a monk, a Guru, who was in retreat in a remote area up in the hills. I would spend the day listening to my friends and Geshe-La converse and debate in Tibetan, catching the odd word. We would all be squeezed into Geshe-La's tiny abode as we sipped hot, salted butter-tea. I hoped that some of the profound teachings that were being shared were filtering into my mind, despite my not understanding most of what was said.

I was well aware that many of the Buddhist teachings that we were gifted with were from a direct lineage passed from teacher to student over many generations. I understood this was precious and rare and would become rarer as the teachings were adapted and spread into our global culture. I have been very blessed to sit at the feet of many masters from the Buddhist tradition and others.

The main work of the hospital was running a tuberculosis-control programme, as this disease was very prevalent amongst Tibetans-in-exile. This gave me the opportunity to travel, in that trusty jeep, to many of the Tibetan settlements in the state of Himachal Pradesh.

Delek Hospital was half way between the town of Dharamsala, at the base of the hills, and the village of McLeod Gang further up the hills. There was a winding mountain road that went from Dharamsala to McLeod Gang. Delek Hospital was perched on the side of this road, about halfway between both towns.

I made the journey up that road by foot many times. There was a teahouse, called 'Devi's Half-Way House', that was further up that road from the hospital. On my way to McLeod Gang I would often stop for a cup of hot chai, and sit on a wooden bench outside that little tearoom overlooking the most spectacular scenery of the Western Himalaya.

The Dalai Lama was my neighbour. His monastery was up the hill from the hospital, in the town of McLeod Gang. That winding road took you almost to the doorstep of his monastery. On occasion he would be driven, in his Range Rover, down that winding road on his way to Delhi and overseas locations.

When word got around that the Dalai Lama might be travelling down to the plains, the hospital's staff, and any patient that could, would run out of the hospital to line the road in the hope of getting a glimpse of His Holiness, and pay reverence to him, as he travelled by. I was one of them and I recall a time when, as he passed us in his vehicle, our eyes met briefly and he gave me his warm, friendly smile and waved. Years later, I would be amongst an audience of thousands in my home city of Melbourne to be in his presence. I have seen that same friendly smile often via his media coverage.

Dharamsala, in the foothills of the Western Himalaya, was a 'hill station'. It was where the British used to go to escape the searing heat of the plains in summer and reside in the cooler and more alpine terrain of the foothills. Remnants of the 'Raj' dotted the area, in contrast to the more traditional Indian and Tibetan buildings. After Indian independence and the 'parturition' most of the British left India; though often their hearts remained in this exotic land that was their home. And some 'stayed on'.

There was such a couple, who lived in a cottage much further up the hills beyond McLeod Gang, whose family had stayed on. They lived in a quintessential English cottage nestled in a remote area high up in the foothills. Their cottage had a white picket fence and a piano took pride of place. Unreachable by road, the piano had been carried up the steep hills by porters. Bear and panthers roamed those hills and legend had it that the couple's little dog was taken by a panther when it had ventured outside that white picket fence.

I never saw a bear in those areas, but I remember one day, when I was alone on duty at the hospital, word got around that a man, who had been attacked by a bear, and apparently with severe injuries, was being carried down to our hospital. Not something I had seen a lot of during my city hospital training. Much to my relief our little hospital was by-passed and the victim was taken to a larger hospital in the plains. Working at Delek Hospital provided me with a number of medical experiences that I would never see in my city training.

Each year, this English couple, who had stayed on, gathered a number of people to celebrate Christmas in their home. This included the visiting staff from Delek Hospital; and this year I was one of them. The idea was to reproduce the traditional Christmas festivities that many of us had grown up with.

We were a motley crew from all over the globe, and most of us had not even met each other prior to that day, yet we were to celebrate Christmas together like we had known each other forever. Travel is like that. Away from our homelands, and past identities, we make quick and deep connections with other people. We did not have to contend with the family dramas that this time of the year can so readily flush up.

This Christmas it snowed. I had arrived in Dharamsala during monsoon, and misty cloud hung low in the sky during all of that season. In those parts monsoon cleared almost overnight. One morning, not long before Christmas, I opened my windows to unexpectedly see a blanket of snow covering the whole area, with the peaks of the Western Himalaya jutting majestically in the distance. It was like the heavens had parted. It was a brilliance to behold.

On Christmas day another volunteer doctor and I trudged up the snow-covered hills to reach the cottage. It was a long journey on foot and we were ill-prepared for the cold but fuelled by anticipation of shared Christmas festivities and a welcome break from our work. I had received a Christmas parcel from home that contained Christmas treats and delicacies, which I took with me as my contribution for the day.

We had a wonderful day as a number of us gathered, ate and drank in this little English cottage high in the hills of North India. We sang around that piano that had been carried up the hills on porter's backs. It was very wonderful and very surreal to be celebrating Christmas in this little cottage, nestled in the snowy foothills of the Western Himalaya.

We stayed overnight, as it would be far too dangerous to travel down the hills at night. The next day, replete with food and festivities, we journeyed down the hills to resume our duties at Delek Hospital. We had said our good-byes to people we knew we might never see again; but with whom we shared a wonderful day, the memory of which would linger for many years.

I would be leaving India soon after that Christmas in the Himalayan foothills, as my term at the hospital was nearly up. I would be going home – though my heart would linger in this exotic land.

I have experienced many Christmases since then, most in my homeland of Australia and one in California. I occasionally think of that 'white Christmas' in India and the many other adventures experienced in that wonderful land. I thank that experience for helping to broaden my worldview.

About the Author

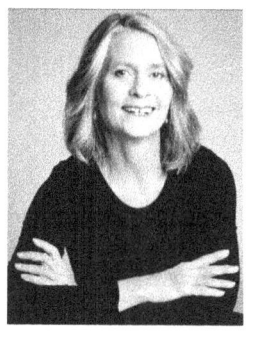

Dr Fyans has been a medical practitioner for over 35 years, graduating from Monash University medical school in 1979. She has a passionate interest in 'mind-body' medicine, particularly in the subconscious-mind influences on physical and psychological health. Her interest in this area was ignited when she worked with Tibetan refugees in North India in the mid-1980s. There she was exposed to another world-view, which for her challenged many of the dogmas that were instilled during her medical training. She gained a greater understanding of the role that mind/consciousness plays in health and all aspects of life.

Her interests led her to study a number of other health-care practises, including kinesiology. She enjoys having a 'foot in both worlds' and this has given her an insight into the spectrum of health-care practises. She continues to practise as an 'integrative' general medical practitioner. Her aim is to combine the best of what these various health-care disciplines have to offer; and bring about a greater understanding of the primacy of mind/consciousness in health, wellbeing and life in general.

She lives near Melbourne, Australia, and her interests include painting, hiking, fitness and metaphysical studies. She is the proud mother of two sons.

www.ingramcontent.com/pod-product-compliance
Lightning Source LLC
LaVergne TN
LVHW011910080426
835508LV00007BA/329